Anterior Segment Repair and Reconstruction:

Techniques and Medico-legal Issues

To Sarah, Mandy and Wendy

Acquisitions editor: Melanie Tait
Development editor: Zoë Youd
Production controller: Chris Jarvis
Desk editor: Jane Campbell
Cover designer: Greg Harris

Anterior Segment Repair and Reconstruction

Techniques and Medico-legal Issues

Bruce A. Noble BSc, FRCS, FRCOphth
Consultant Ophthalmologist and
Director of Anterior Segment Service,
United Leeds Teaching Hospitals, Leeds, UK
Senior Clinical Lecturer in Ophthalmology,
Leeds University Department of Surgery, Leeds, UK

Ian G. Simmons BVSc, MB, ChB, FRCS, FRCOphth
Consultant Ophthalmologist,
United Leeds Teaching Hospitals, Leeds, UK
Senior Clinical Lecturer in Ophthalmology,
Leeds University Department of Science, Leeds, UK

Bernard Y. P. Chang BSC, MB, ChB, FRCSEd, FRCOphth
Specialist Registrar,
The General Infirmary at Leeds, Leeds, UK

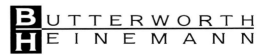

OXFORD AUCKLAND BOSTON JOHANNESBURG MELBOURNE NEW DELHI

Butterworth-Heinemann
Linacre House, Jordan Hill, Oxford OX2 8DP
225 Wildwood Avenue, Woburn, MA 01801-2041
A division of Reed Educational and Professional Publishing Ltd

℞ A member of the Reed Elsevier plc group

First published 2002

British Library Cataloguing in Publication Data
Noble, Bruce A.
    Anterior segment repair and reconstruction: techniques and medico–legal issues
    1.   Anterior segment (Eye) – Surgery
    I.   Title   II.   Simmons, Ian G.   III.   Chang, Bernard Y.P.
    617.7'1

Library of Congress Cataloguing in Publication Data
A catalogue record for this book is available from the Library of Congress

ISBN 0 7506 4573 3

For information on all Butterworth-Heinemann publications visit our website at www.bh.com

Designed, Illustrated and Typeset by Keyword Typesetting Services Ltd, Wallington Surrey
Printed and bound in Italy

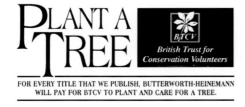

FOR EVERY TITLE THAT WE PUBLISH, BUTTERWORTH-HEINEMANN
WILL PAY FOR BTCV TO PLANT AND CARE FOR A TREE.

Contents

Preface

This book sets out to challenge the *laissez-faire* attitude to complications and injuries. Faced with a damaged eye, perhaps as a result of your own surgical complication, what are you going to do? Do you ignore the problem, deny its presence or allow its management to drift 'down' the clinic for the clinical assistant to muffle the patient's dismay? Is there anything that can be done, and if so, can you do it? Are your plans for surgical reconstruction safe or wise and do they reflect a need to appease your ego rather than to improve your patient's quality of life?

'Anterior segment reconstruction' is not a term usually found indexed in a textbook of ophthalmic surgery. The reason for this is that it isn't just one single surgical procedure, but rather a synthesis of many microsurgical techniques that are used together to restore the structure, appearance and function of an eye. The multiple steps are used together or in a programme of operations, each contributing to the final function. Whether eyes have been damaged previously by accident, assault or surgery, the intuitive application of appropriate techniques can give these damaged eyes a chance of a permanent, comfortable vision.

In a perfect world there would be neither eye injuries nor complications of surgery requiring corrective treatment. But accidents, military mutilations and surgical disasters continue and even though the techniques for cataract surgery have got safer, a steady yield of patients needing surgical restoration of their eyes continues. Every new technique has a learning curve; with every learning curve comes a new harvest of complications. Previously, such damage was a sentence to pain and poor vision for the patient, but the tools and microsurgical techniques developed in the past 30 years have improved the possible outcomes for these patients. Microscopes, sutures, microinstrumentation, vitreous techniques, viscoelastics and intraocular lenses have all played their part in advancing the cause of ophthalmology.

Anterior segment reconstruction, then, is the synthesis of these many methods, used together, at the same time or in a logical order, to permanently restore sight to severely damaged eyes. Nearly all of these surgical steps should be in the common repertoire of any ophthalmic surgeon. For example, following complicated surgery some months previously, an eye reveals a dislocated intraocular lens, vitreous incarcerated in the wound, hiding behind a cornea, opaque with oedema. Lens explantation, secondary implantation, vitrectomy and keratoplasty will all be needed to repair this eye. The operations may be done simultaneously or in series of steps at different times. Similarly, the logical application of combined biological and surgical techniques allows restoration of the ocular surface after a chemical injury.

Who should read the book? It is our intention that the techniques of primary repair, the principles of management of surgical complications and secondary reconstruction are described in such a way as to be accessible for any surgeon, of any level, who is operating on their own or supervising juniors. Our aim has been to devise a practical and direct, bench-top manual. This is based on 20 years' experience of undertaking anterior segment surgery, and training and teaching microsurgery to trainees of various levels of experience. The text is illustrated with drawings, digitally-captured per-operative images and slit-lamp photographs. We have used drawings as a way of more clearly showing the technique and subtleties of the surgery; drawings should convey how things appear to the surgeon. There are, of course, many alternative ways of doing these operations; we acknowledge this but show those that in our hands have proved reliable.

When should you read the book? The information presented in the first section of the book should be thought of as core knowledge and should be readily available as a bench-top book to help any surgeon (often of registrar level) repair a damaged eye. The second section can be used for reference purposes, to help plan an elective reconstruction. To make it easier to use, individual points are not referenced in the text but a list of recommended reading has been included towards the back of the book. Weightier tomes discuss all the available options for each step along the treatment path. This book has been designed to be more didactic, offering practical advice from an extensive experience.

The third section of the book deals with the special cases of damage to a child's eye, chemical injuries and patient-handling problems. A separate chapter has been devoted to the approaches to specific paediatric problems rather than lacing these throughout the rest of the book. The ocular surface is a new domain, and the strategies for restoring the ocular surface in these damaged eyes are set out so as to provide a logical approach to this new arena of therapy.

The last section deals with the difficult issues of litigation. There is an economic and human cost for every injury and every surgical accident. As surgeons, we will be involved in any of several processes of law. Whether operating, advising a patient or a lawyer, or defending yourself or a colleague, a knowledge of the principles of the law of personal injury is invaluable. Similarly knowledge of the possible outcomes for surgery (the 'evidence base') should be known or available to justify or explain to patients (and/or lawyers). We were extremely fortunate to have had the advice and scholarship of Mr James Goss Q.C., who read and criticised our legalese. As a result, we hope that this chapter is up to date, relevant and useful for both doctors and lawyers alike.

We hope that these two chapters will stimulate further reading into this unfortunately growing speciality; and that the tables of disability and probability of outcomes will prove useful to our legal colleagues.

Acknowledgements

The patience and support of our colleagues have been crucial. In particular, we are grateful to the following who read or commented on our efforts; Prof. Doug Coster, who looked critically at the chapter on the ocular surface; Piers Percival for his advice on the treatment of astigmatism; Robert Doran, who pulled our chapter on paediatrics into a clearer focus; Colin Vize, Raymond Loh and Anita Reynolds who read and critiqued and provided editorial commentary. Keith Clarke of Ethicon Ltd, Glyne Allen of Vision Matrix, Hong Woon and Stephen Spencer all loaned us slides and we thank them for their help. The consultant pathologists of neuro- and ocular pathology, in the Leeds University Department of Pathology, have provided long-term support and their photographic studies of unusual cases are well used in the book. We are also grateful to Bernard Garstang who made available to us the important document on quantification of disability after visual injuries. Drs Jenny Burr and Paul Brogden have worked in our anterior segment clinic for many years and they have supported this work and the patients who underwent the surgery, playing that crucial role ensuring human and visual success for all the surgical effort. Their criticisms have helped us greatly.

We must pick out the special efforts of Mr Tim Henderson FRCOphth, who read the book through in its multiple early drafts, and whose criticism and enthusiasm helped us clarify our thoughts. To John Gibson, anaesthetist and friend, we owe particular thanks for his calm support as we developed or practised these techniques, or taught them to our juniors. Mike Geall, Principal Medical Photographer, took most of the slides for us. The most difficult images to capture in ophthalmology are those of the anterior segment, and we admire his efforts and persistence over the past 20 years. Our diagrams and drawings have been processed into superb illustrations by Kim Barrance. His ability to take simple sketches and turn them into finished, fresh drawings has been so important in helping us convey our ideas to our readers. We are especially grateful to him.

We would like to thank Sisters Sue Boyes and Pat Clark and their team in the eye theatre at Leeds General Infirmary. Their intuitive assistance during complex operations was never more clearly demonstrated than when after they had been asked time and again, for a particular instrument, they would unfailingly place in your hand what was needed rather than what had been 'asked for'! Colin Osbourne and his team at LIMIT (Leeds Institute for Minimally Invasive Therapy) were instrumental in the production of the digitally-captured operative images.

The help of Caroline Makepeace, Melanie Tait, Zoë Youd and their team at Butterworth-Heinemann has made the difficult transition from scribbled notes to finished article possible and enjoyable.

Finally our wives deserve a special mention, as do the spouses of all medical authors who struggle to accept the ever-increasing clinical and writing burdens into already-overfull schedules. Again, this book is dedicated to them.

Abbreviations

ABK	Aphakic bullous keratopathy	KLAL	Keratolimbal allografting
AC	Anterior chamber	LAL	Limbal allograft
ACGR	Australian Corneal Graft Registry	LAU	Limbal autografting
A&E	Accident and emergency	LI	Limbal ischaemia
AISH	Acute intraoperative suprachoroidal haemmorhage	LSC	Limbal stem cell
		LSCD	Limbal stem cell deficiency
AM	Amniotic membrane	LSG	Limbal stem cell graft
AMT	Amniotic membrane transplantation	MRI	Magnetic resonance imaging
ARMD	Age-related macula degeneration	MVR	Micro-vitreo-retinal
ATR	Against-the-rule	MW	Molecular weight
BMA	British Medical Association	NAI	Non-accidental injury
BSS	Balanced salt solution	NCSS	National Cataract Surgery Survey
CCC	Continuous curvilinear capsulorrhexis	Nd:YAG	Neodymium: yttrium, aluminium, garnet
CF	Counting fingers	NPL	No perception of light
CMO	Cystoid macular oedema	OS	Ocular surface
CSP	Common starting point	OSD	Ocular surface disease
CT	Computerized tomography	OSR	Ocular surface reconstruction
DFN	Dalen–Fuchs nodules	PBK	Pseudophakic bullous keratopathy
DVLA	Driving and Vehicle Licensing Agency	PC	Posterior chamber
ECCE	Extracapsular cataract extraction	PCC	Professional Conduct Committee
FBC	Full blood count	PCO	Posterior capsular opacification
FCT	Fluorescein clearance test	PED	Persistent epithelial defect
GA	General anaesthesia	PKP	Penetrating keratoplasty
GMC	General Medical Council	PL	Perception of light
HGV	Heavy goods vehicle	PMMA	Polymethylmethacrylate
HM	Hand movements	PPCCC	Primary posterior capsulorrhexis
HSM	Heparin-surface modification	RAPD	Relative afferent pupillary defect
ICCE	Intracapsular cataract extraction	RD	Retinal detachment
ICL	Implantable contact lens	RPE	Retinal pigment epithelium
IOFB	Intraocular foreign body	SO	Sympathetic ophthalmia
IOL	Intraocular lens	TGFβ	Transforming growth factor β
IOP	Intraocular pressure	VA	Visual acuity
IV	Intravenous	WTR	With-the-rule

Repair and Recovery

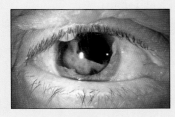

1 The common starting point and the therapeutic plan

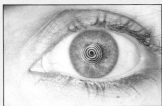

2 Primary response – the principles of management of surgical complications and the repair of ocular injuries

Chapter 1

The common starting point and the therapeutic plan

INTRODUCTION

An early audit in Leeds of 100 consecutive anterior segment reconstructions showed that more than 55 per cent were due to insults resulting from the complications of cataract surgery and 45 per cent to accidental and criminal trauma. Traumatic cases may be more dramatic as they present via emergency rooms, but of equal relevance in this study was the damage, not always immediately recognized, following surgery. Although the success rate of lens surgery is excellent, we dare not forget that the most frequent wound made in an eye is the incision for removal of a cataract. Moreover, it is possible for surgical interference with the eye to seed a series of problems as damaging as overt injury from extraneous other causes. Even local variations in the statistic quoted cannot invalidate the relevance of this retrospective analysis.

ROUTES TO THE COMMON STARTING POINT

Eye injuries cover the gamut of human experience from the trivial to the critical. Each wreaks its own havoc on the globe, orbit, or adnexa. The traumatic cases present acutely and then receive appropriate surgical repair in the operating theatre to try to save the eye. The need for the surgical interference is accepted by the patient who hopes not to lose sight. Consequently, patients are more receptive of a poor outcome knowing that the doctor has 'done their best' and is therefore the 'hero'.

On the other hand, severe and blinding events can also occur during routine surgery which has been undertaken to restore, not remove, sight. For instance, in a cataract operation, the hopes of the patient will be dashed when their elective operation can only be completed after complicated surgery. Furthermore, if, when the complication occurs, the handling of this is inadequate, the post-operative progress will be marked by a procession of visits through the clinics over months and years. If the pathological signs are ignored the patient is damned to a dismal ocular future. Despite appropriate management of a complication, if the visual outcome is poor, the doctor will be perceived as the 'villain'.

Figure 1.1 shows an eye which had a vitrectomy following a capsule tear during cataract surgery; Fig. 1.2 shows an eye injured by a criminal assault with a broken bottle. In both there has been loss of iris tissue; in both, fragments of lens and capsule occlude the pupil. The end-results of both scenarios are very similar. Both cases pose problems to the surgeon of how to repair and restore sight.

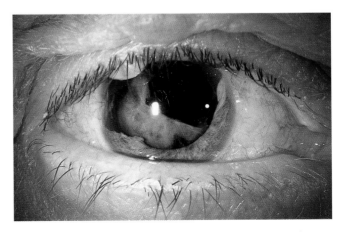

Figure 1.1. An eye following a complicated cataract operation.

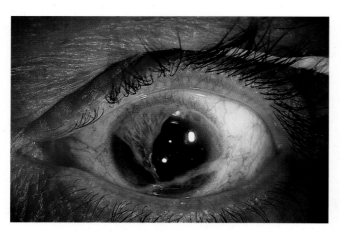

Figure 1.2. An eye injured with a broken bottle.

The nature and severity of the insult, and the scarring response of the eye to the trauma, will decide the final outcome for any particular eye. At worst, the eye will be blind and painful; in others, corneal damage, scarring, vitreous incarceration, distorted pupil and capsular membranes may be present. Retinal damage, contusion, perforation, detachment or macular oedema, perhaps hidden by opacities in the media, will further complicate and affect the visual outcome. Prompt, skilful surgical treatment can temper the outcome in the same way that appropriate handling of a surgical complication will reduce adverse sequelae.

Scheme 1.1 indicates two possible routes which may follow an ocular insult. From the instant of trauma or a surgical complication, a cascade of problems and opportunities flows to an end-point which may leave an eye requiring further surgical intervention to restore function, comfort or appearance. This common pathological end-point becomes the common starting point (CSP) for surgical reconstruction.

Ocular trauma

The visual outcome of ocular trauma depends on the nature, extent and cause of the injury and on the ocular structures involved. The more posterior the structure involved, the more complex the injury and, often, the poorer the outcome. The trauma may be penetrating, blunt or chemical.

Unlike a surgical complication, where the surgeon is present at the time of the injury and has the chance to treat, limit or modify the process, accidental injuries happen rapidly and cannot be contained or treated until the patient reaches the clinic. Their extent is limited only by chance and the nature of the insult. In the accident and emergency (A&E) department, triage will identify a serious problem but it will only be when the patient has been seen by an ophthalmologist that preparations for surgical repair can be started. There then follows a delay, often a matter of hours, before definitive treatment can be given. (The evolution of a chemical injury can be greatly modified by good first aid and prompt treatment in the A&E department, in anticipation of more extended treatment protocols if the injury is serious.) Opportunities for secondary treatment, whether surgical or optical, will present in the days, weeks and months after the primary injury.

It is important that the quality of the primary repair, whether simple suturing or complex intervention, is of the highest quality. The possibilities of reconstruction are limited by the quality of the primary repair and the state of the tissues that remain in the eye. The more 'normal' the anatomy remains, the greater the options for further advanced surgery.

Surgical complications

There are two alternative pathways for an elective operation such as cataract surgery, complicated or uncomplicated. The pathway (Scheme 1.1) following a surgical complication is a challenge both immediately and later when reconstructive management may be needed. The indicated pathway follows the evolution of a complication. It can be seen that the surgeon has a series of opportunities to recover and improve the outcome; these may be either during or after the operation. At all times, the quality of the surgical and medical response will directly influence the visual outcome. If clumsily or inadequately handled, the reconstructive challenge (if ever offered) is more difficult, and has a less certain outcome. For example, pseudophakic bullous keratopathy is frequently associated with chronic cystoid macular oedema; a uniformly poor outcome is to be expected unless there is early re-intervention.

The alternative pathway, that of competently and safely completed surgery, needs no further comment. The structural and visual objectives will have been safely reached.

FORWARD PLANNING

The common starting point is the pathological problem that needs correction, revision or reconstruction. Both the affected eye and the patient as a whole must be considered, and when all the information is collated a plan can be formulated. Such a 'plan' may seem rather grandiose if the problem is small, but in an increasingly litigious world, any thought-processes and agreements between yourself and your patient must be carefully documented.

Chapter 2

Primary response – the principles of management of surgical complications and the repair of ocular injuries

MANAGING SURGICAL COMPLICATIONS

Introduction

The emphasis of this section is on the 'principles' of management of the complications of anterior segment surgery and in particular, phakoemulsification (phaco) cataract surgery; the detailed technical steps are presented in our companion volume *Complications of Cataract Surgery: A Manual*. Similarly, because corneal and glaucoma surgery is increasingly undertaken by specialists, the details of these operative techniques belong to more dedicated tomes and will consequently only be covered in passing.

When we reviewed 50 consecutive patients referred to us for complex secondary surgery, over 90 per cent of those who had complications at their primary operation were undergoing cataract surgery at the time, and in all of these vitreous had been 'lost'. This is not in itself surprising when so many cataract operations are undertaken every year. At presentation the pathology observed included corneal decompensation, iris tethering and loss, ill-placed intraocular lenses (IOLs), uveitis and glaucoma. In the posterior segment, retinal detachment and cystoid macula oedema were seen. Pain and poor vision were the common, unifying, symptoms.

At this review, it was clear that better handling of the initial complication would have avoided poor visual out-comes and the need for surgical revision. In many of the cases, it also appeared that the primary problem had not been recognized at the original operation or had gone unrecognized at the post-operative visits. Thus the problems were allowed to persist and the secondary effects to develop, resulting in irrecoverable damage. The common surgical misadventure (of vitreous loss), married to the recurring failure to properly manage this complication, denied these patients a good outcome.

When vitreous is left incarcerated around structures in the anterior chamber, it will bind, drag, displace and pull. Pain and poor vision are symptomatic of the resulting intraocular inflammation and damage. Delay compounds the problems, and yet the rules of management are straight-forward. With modern instrumentation, and appropriate intervention, a quite different outcome can be expected. Anticipation of risk, good procedures, trained staff and a clear understanding of the technique and purpose of the surgical steps should see a good visual result for that eye. The need for secondary surgery will then be reduced and, if required, undertaken in a timely way and without the confounding effects of the secondary pathological changes.

Any surgical mishap threatens the visual recovery of the eye. No surgeon is exempt, beginner or master. What separates a good from a bad operator is how they manage complications (it could be argued a surgeon's quality should be judged by their ability to handle complications).

In cataract surgery, as in any routine operation, the successful completion of one step lets you proceed to the next step as planned. Equally, however, a problem, however small, will impinge on subsequent steps exponentially worsening the situation. Alternative strategies will be required. You have to be able to not only know how to do the standard operation, but also know what to do when something goes wrong. To be able to respond appropriately to a complication you have to know what alternative routes out of trouble were available when the problem began. This 'knowledge' must be instinctively available; it cannot be learned by just reading books but needs practical application. The only way to attain these skills is by actual surgical experience and, in turn, that experience can only be acquired by spending many hours watching, assisting and performing surgery.

Prevention

The conventional view is that if a complication occurs, it is the fault of the surgeon. Of course, nothing can replace the golden principles that make sound technique, good instrumentation and rigorous attention to detail the cornerstones of high-quality surgery. Failure to deliver on this account is indefensible. In cataract surgery, especially phaco, safe practice depends on a series of different factors including staff training and protocols, the performance characteristics of the machinery, an understanding of the fluid dynamics and careful case selection. Structured surgical training underpins the acquisition of good surgical habits, including operating posture, and must be matched by insight into one's limitations.

However, a broader overview is also needed, because not every surgical complication is the result of a surgeon's mistake. For instance when a case develops endophthalmitis the problem could have started at any one of several stages of the operation. Alternatively and more importantly, if there have been a series of disasters, any one of the many steps in the process of management may be pivotal. This includes poor surgical scrub technique, manufacturing contamination of fluids, faults in sterilization of instruments, and a change of supplier and product (e.g. to an apparently cheaper alternative).

To establish the cause, the whole 'system' has to be scrutinized. With so many people, actions and steps involved in running an operating list, contamination could have happened at any of several stages. Good practice demands that there are appropriate checks in the system to prevent such disasters from happening, and to enable back-checking if problems occur. It is essential practice to maintain records of all staff, instruments, fluids, batch numbers, dressings and drugs used for each and every case. Remember that not every problem is apparent on the operating table, and that late, sometimes very late, presentation of infection or corneal damage can occur. In these cases, the process of backtracking is only possible if there is a system in place which fastidiously records all details as routine.

To claim that your role is solely that of 'surgeon' is naïve. Certainly there is a narrow defile of activity for which you are directly responsible and accountable, but there is also a wider, joint responsibility, shared with senior theatre staff, to maintain an overview of the whole process of surgery. Every member of the theatre team is a stakeholder in its safe practices, but as surgeon, your participation in overseeing the whole system is a fundamental role. With this perspective, the whole process can be fully explored.

Skills required to manage complications

The surgeon must be able to cope with the complications of any operation they start or supervise. Certain core skills are needed and those for phacoemulsificaton are listed in Table 2.1. The challenge when something goes wrong during an operation is to escape without doing more damage. It may be better to close the eye if the patient is unsatisfactorily mobile during the operation. Ask for help from a colleague if the problem is beyond your grasp.

A complication will often begin in a small way, e.g. a radial tear of the capsule. If this snag is ignored or you fail to adapt your approach to the case, the tear will extend. This may result in the loss of nuclear fragments into the vitreous, and the prolapse of vitreous through the rent into the anterior chamber. The problem will increase in its extent and threat, the longer it goes unnoticed. As in a penetrating injury, where a good repair makes for a better outcome, an appropriate surgical response to a per-operative complication similarly improves the prognosis for the eye. If the tissues are handled carefully and in particular if the vitreous is cleared from the pupil and wound, it should be possible to complete the operation and achieve an excellent visual result (Table 2.2).

Each technique needs experience and detailed study to understand the nuances of how to respond.

The core skills required to manage the complications of cataract surgery are presented in detail in our companion volume. It is of some concern that current surgical teaching

Table 2.1. Core skills in the management of the surgical complications of cataract surgery.
Techniques for conversion from phacoemulsification to extracapsular cataract surgery.
Handling capsular tears and use of any capsular remnants.
Alternative ways of removing the lens or remnants after a tear in the capsule.
Recognizing vitreous prolapse and how to do an anterior vitrectomy.
Implantation of an IOL when the routine methods of support are no longer available.
Suturing wounds.
Managing a supra-choroidal haemorrhage (see Table 2.2).
Post-operative care of eyes and patients having had complicated surgery.

Table 2.2. Managing acute supra-choroidal haemorrhage.

Incidence	0.2–0.9% of cataract operations	
Risk factors	Increased axial length	
	Raised intra-ocular pressure	
Types	Expulsive	spontaneous nucleus expression with extrusion of ocular contents
	Non-expulsive	supra-choroidal haemorrhage without loss of ocular contents
Signs	Shallowing of the anterior chamber, loss of the red reflex, extrusion of ocular contents and prolapse of the iris. The majority of AISH occurs after removal of the nucleus.	
Actions	Immediate	Close the wound quickly and tightly (8-0 or thicker suture material may be required)
		Perform posterior sclerotomies (1.5 mm in diameter) if the eye cannot be closed
	Later	Wait for the clot of any massive haemorrhage to liquefy (which takes 3–5 days) and then drain with posterior sclerotomies under constant infusion pressure. Treat any retinal detachment as indicated
Outcomes	Around 33 per cent will require a secondary surgical procedure	
	20 per cent will attain a post-operative vision of 6/12 or better	
	A poor visual outcome of CF or worse is often seen where there has been spontaneous nuclear expression or where vision is only PL at first dressing.	
	A favourable visual outcome is more common with AISH complicating phacoemulsification as opposed to standard extra-capsular surgery (this is probably due to the speed of wound closure with consequent containment of the haemorrhage).	

rarely gives the trainees the opportunity to perform an extracapsular cataract extraction (ECCE). Phaco is actually a form of extracapsular surgery but we have left the terms 'phaco' and 'ECCE' as the distinct entities. This means that the techniques of nuclear expression, knowledge of how to use the irrigating vectis and to suture a wound are becoming unrehearsed. These same skills are needed to handle the complications of phacoemulsification. Efforts are needed to acquire and teach these additional skills, which are not usually part of the syllabus of a phaco course.

Because of its common relevance to both reconstructive surgery and the complications of cataract surgery, we will discuss the approach to vitreous loss in the next section.

Vitreous loss and anterior vitrectomy

Vitreous, so silent in the posterior segment, assumes an altogether different, almost aggressive role in the anterior segment, with many undesirable effects. The release of vitreous occurs when the protective wall of the lens capsule is damaged. Once inundation of the anterior segment occurs, a trail of undesirable effects becomes possible (see Table 2.3).

Some of these may seem unrelated to the presentation of vitreous into the anterior chamber (AC), but on reflection, it is readily seen that the surgical manipulations will have taken longer and caused corneal endothelial damage. Infection is more likely to occur because of the extended surgical time, if vitreous is incarcerated in the larger wound, and especially if tissues have been macerated. Vitreous binds the iris, lens and capsule together and entangles any IOL, pulling the pupil into bizarre shapes and displacing the IOL. Normal iris movement is restricted and this finding is associated with a marked and chronic

Table 2.3. Possible pathological consequences of vitreous loss during anterior segment surgery.

Uveitis
Glaucoma
Inaccurate placing of the IOL
Endophthalmitis
Cystoid macular oedema
Retinal detachment
Bullous keratopathy

iritis. Unless the iris is freed from these restraining bonds, this inflammation will not resolve.

When vitreous becomes incarcerated, the retina and the anterior segment are physically linked together. Anterior–posterior traction pulls on the vitreous base or peripheral retina causing retinal tears and detachment of the retina; cystoid macular oedema can also result if the traction is unrelieved and is aggravated by coexisting uveitis. The patient will complain of pain and poor vision.

These pathological processes are initially reversible, but with time the secondary effects become chronic and intractable. Secondary glaucoma, bullous keratopathy and cystoid macular oedema are difficult to treat, with at best modest visual outcomes. Delay makes it hard, if not impossible, to put things right.

PRINCIPLES OF ANTERIOR VITRECTOMY

If vitreous presents during anterior segment surgery, it must be completely cleared from the structures at the front of the eye. This is a fundamental skill that every ophthalmic surgeon should master. Variations on the method will be determined by the actual stage of the operation reached, and limited by the instruments available. If you feel comfortable with the method and its purpose, then the complication of capsule rupture and vitreous loss will always be competently handled. Familiarity in the use and setting up of vitreous cutting machinery is mandatory. Both surgical and theatre support staff must be able to promptly play their part if and when a vitrectomy is required in the anterior segment.

A good vitreous cutter is essential to avoid retinal traction and to complete the clearance of the anterior segment. It is dangerous to merely swab the surgical wound with sponges and cut away the presenting strands with scissors. It is rarely effective in ensuring complete removal or clearance from the anterior segment.

Use low bottle-height for the infusion. Check that there is sufficient flow into the anterior chamber so that it can be maintained whilst aspirating. When performing the vitrectomy, endeavour to draw the vitreous backwards, away from the AC, into the posterior segment, completely clearing the pupil margin and anterior chamber. The surgery should be limited to this simple objective. It should be done carefully and gently, avoiding damaging the iris and capsule, remembering that it is dangerous to attempt any surgery in the posterior segment beyond clearing the pupillary plane.

A separate infusion is preferable, passed through a paracentesis, e.g. use a butterfly cannula held in artery forceps (see Figs 2.1a and b). When an infusion sleeve around the vitrector is used, the balanced salt solution (BSS) will be directed into the vitreous, encouraging further prolapse. The bottle-height of the infusion should be moderate to low or vitreous will be impelled into the anterior chamber and through the wound, compounding the problem.

TECHNIQUE (see Fig 2.2)

As the problem becomes obvious and you suspect that the vitreous is beginning to come forward into the AC, ask the nursing staff to prepare for a vitrectomy. Immediately lower the height of the infusion bottle to reduce the intraocular pressure but keep the instruments in the eye.

Prevent fragments of lens or cortex from tumbling backwards with a probe or second instrument. Slowly remove the phaco probe and reform the anterior chamber with viscoelastic, which can also be used to help plug the posterior capsular defect, keeping nuclear fragments in the anterior segment. The most common time for posterior capsule rupture to occur is during aspiration, especially for trainees. The use of a dispersive viscoelastic can help tamponade the vitreous back, allowing completion of this step of the operation.

Enlarge the second incision, angling the knife towards the inner opening of the phaco stab. This gives easier access to lens fragments and any vitreous incarcerated into the incision. Insert an infusion cannula into the second incision (e.g. Butterfly 19G. IV cannula), with the bottle-height at approximately 25 cm above the level of the eye, directing the flow of BSS over the iris surface but 'away' from the capsular hole. If the BSS is directed into

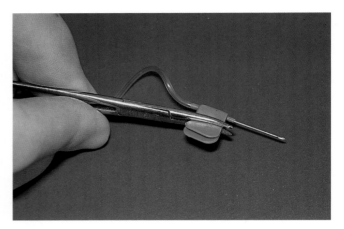

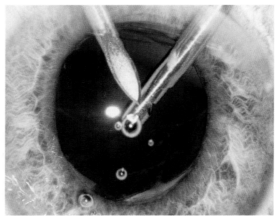

Figure 2.1. (a) Infusion cannula for anterior vitrectomy – a butterfly cannula is held by Spencer Wells forceps. (b) The butterfly cannula used with a vitrector inside the anterior chamber.

the vitreous, it will encourage further prolapse as the fluid mixes with the vitreous.

Remove the lens remnants, cortex, nucleus or capsular shreds as they present to the cutter, but be careful to conserve iris and capsule. The capsulorrhexis must be saved if possible because it will be invaluable for lens implantation.

Feed any remaining lens matter into the port of the vitrector (if the lens matter is either soft or mostly cortical there should be no difficulty). Then pass the cutter through the rent in the capsule and into the anterior vitreous. Using a cutting speed of approximately 360 cuts per minute, aspirate and cut the vitreous, drawing it back from the anterior chamber. If soft nuclear fragments are lost into the posterior segment, do not chase them because they usually come forward into the anterior chamber as the vitrectomy proceeds, stirred up by the turbulence of the infusion. They can be removed as they re-present.

Continue until the anterior segment is clear of vitreous. Check this by passing a probe carefully around the pupil margin, and always recheck the primary incision because vitreous is inevitably found there. Change the angle of the

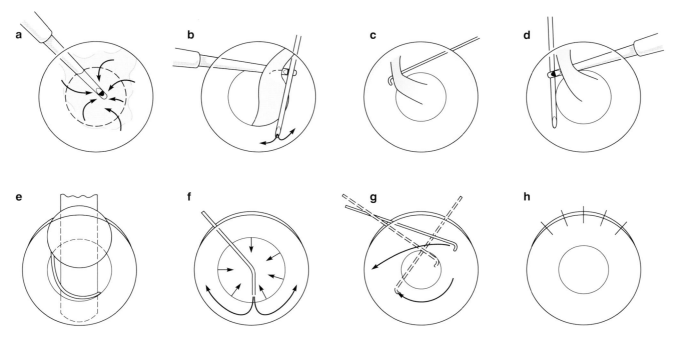

Figure 2.2. Technique of anterior vitrectomy. Note that the vitrector is passed through the pupil into the posterior chamber and the vitreous is sucked and cut, pulling it backwards, from the AC. A separate infusion prevents vitreous hydration and allows individual strands to be identified and cut. The instruments should be interchanged enabling the last strands to be cut.

vitrector or better still reintroduce it through the other port to get a better angle of approach to the region of the inner opening of the wound.

The continuous curvilinear capsulorrhexis (CCC) should be left untouched. It will later provide the means of securing a sulcus-fixated IOL. Check that all surfaces in the anterior segment are free of vitreous. Do this by passing a hook gently across the iris surface and close to the internal opening of the eye and looking for tugging on the pupil margin. Visualization of strands is improved by filling the anterior chamber with air.

Reverse the probes again and check the stab incision. No movement of the pupil margin should be seen, indicating that the AC is free of vitreous. Inject acetylcholine (Miochol, CIBA Vision Ophthalmics) to constrict the pupil and look for peaking of the pupil. If this is found it indicates that there is still more vitreous that needs to be tidied up. Repeat the steps until the pupil margin is clear.

The incision is now opened to allow the implantation of an IOL, the further details of which are discussed in our companion volume.

Post-operative management

In any eye that has had a surgical complication, the aim is to reduce inflammatory sequelae and to prevent a marked pressure rise. Acetozolamide (250 mg) is given routinely immediately after surgery, in the absence of contra-indications. The patient should be seen the next day by a member of the surgical team and told what had happened. Topical steroids are given in increased frequency and strength, matched to the slit-the lamp findings. Further acetozolamide (250 mg, four times a day) is given if the intraocular pressure (IOP) is high and should be continued for two or three days until the pressure is stabilized and normal.

Patient management

Before agreeing to any operation, a patient should have been briefed as to the sort of surgery they were to undergo, and have been told the likelihood of success or complications to be expected.

If there is a complication during or following surgery, the sooner the patient is informed of the problem the better. At the very least they will have to be submitted to further or more extended treatment. If the problem is only noted at a routine clinic visit later on, the patient needs to be told immediately of the problem. Encourage the patient to bring a friend or relative if the news is bad, or the issue complicated. It has been shown time and again that this sort of straightforward relationship with the patient helps both surgeon and patient when things go wrong, and recruits their involvement in their problems.

Medico-legal issues are important and litigation must always be a possibility in any medical contact. By maintaining the highest medical standards, the chances of such a case going to law being successful are reduced; keep accurate, contemporary notes, talk to the patient, encourage them to ask questions, answer their questions in a manner that you think they will understand, and without patronizing them. Keep up to date with your continuing professional development, and be able to prove that you actively participate in audit.

TRAUMA AND PRIMARY REPAIR

Introduction

After any ophthalmic injury it is important to obtain an accurate and fully documented history to establish the cause. Your subsequent examination will identify its extent and the resulting impact on vision. Thoroughness is repaid later when planning treatment and if the injuries are part of legal proceedings. Simple, non-penetrating injuries may be handled as ambulatory cases, whilst more serious injuries need in-patient attention. If surgical repair is needed, per-operative examination will define the extent of that surgery.

Different types of trauma demand different responses and these will be discussed, together with suggested ways of repairing the trauma.

Pre-operative assessment

HISTORY

The patient's perception of their injury should be recorded. Dates, times and the involvement of third parties or occupational equipment should be carefully noted, bearing in mind that such information may be needed for a court case in the distant future (see Table 2.4). It is important to know the nature of the object causing the injury as dirty, organic instruments can inoculate the deeper ocular tissues with less common organisms, such as *Bacillus* spp. and fungi. The patient should be questioned about his tetanus status. The patient's previous ocular history should be recorded including any prior injuries, amblyopia, refractive error or strabismus.

EXAMINATION

A detailed, systematic examination of the eye's function and structure should be performed. This should include visual acuities, with and without a pinhole (and with a pinhole and +10 dioptre lens where there is aphakia). You need to decide whether the eye has any potential to be saved or not, i.e. is the goal a visual or tectonic result? Optic nerve (pupillary reactions) and retinal (light projection) function should be noted even in eyes too damaged to record a visual acuity.

Eyelid, extraocular muscle or orbital injuries should be suspected and looked for in cases of more extensive

Table 2.4. History taking in medico-legal cases.

Demographic data
Patient's name, address, age, date of birth, address and occupation
Date of incident
Date of examination
Examining doctor

Incident/previous surgery
Time, date and place of incident
Third-party and police involvement (any litigation in process)
Previous medical interventions with medical staff names
Current ophthalmic and systemic complaints
Effect of any problems on employment, hobbies and day-to-day living
Patient's perception of his/her disability

General details
Past ocular history (pre-existing amblyopia, strabismus, glaucoma, etc.)
Past medical history including current medications
Current and past employment (including time off work)
Hobbies
Social history (e.g. does the patient care for an infirmed relative?)

trauma. Small wounds in the eyelids may appear innocuous but may be entry wounds for penetrating or perforating objects. If such trauma is discovered, penetration by a foreign body should be suspected until confirmed otherwise. One intraocular foreign body does not preclude a second. If possible, all injuries should be recorded photographically, including peri-ocular lesions and those distant to the eyes.

Ocular or cranial injuries can lead to ocular motor dysfunction. Third, fourth or sixth cranial neuropathy will result in an incommitant strabismus. Head trauma can also cause concomitant squints including both eso- and exo-deviations as well as convergence insufficiency and spasm of the near reflex.

Ocular or orbital trauma may extend out of the confines of the orbit into the sinuses or brain. You should have a low threshold for involving colleagues from other specialities such as diagnostic radiology (to help look for a foreign body with X-ray or computerized tomography (CT) scan), neurology and neurosurgery.

The important question to be able to answer pre-operatively (crucial from a patient-consent perspective and in terms of medico-legal justification) is whether the eye has any potential for sight at all. Those eyes with no potential for vision should be enucleated to reduce the small risk of developing sympathetic ophthalmia (see Table 2.5). If possible, obtain a second opinion before enucleation.

Blunt trauma

Blunt injuries cause sudden distraction of the tissues and damage is seen as hyphaema, iris sphincter tears and lens subluxation. Posterior segment signs include commotio retinae, choroidal rupture and giant retinal tears. When

Table 2.5. Sympathetic ophthalmia.

Incidence	Sympathetic ophthalmia (SO) complicates 0.2–0.5% of non-surgical trauma and 0.01 per cent of vitrectomies or retinal detachment procedures. It may also complicate cyclocryotherapy, laser cryoablation and laser photocoagulation.
Presentation	80 per cent of cases occur within three months of the initial insult. SO is a bilateral granulomatous, panuveitis with an insidious onset of pain, photophobia and decreased vision. Initially, the traumatized (exciting) eye is affected followed by the fellow (sympathizing) eye.
	Signs include mutton-fat keratic precipitates, aqueous cells and flare, synechiae, vitreous haze, optic nerve-head oedema and Dalen–Fuchs nodules (DFN) which are yellowish-white spots at the level of the retinal pigment epithelium.
	A few patients may have the extraocular signs more associated with Vogt–Koyanagi–Harada syndrome (hearing problems, vertigo, etc.)
	23–46% of SO cases may be associated with phako-anaphylaxis.
Immunology	There may be an increased frequency of HLA-A11, HLA-DR4 and DRw53.
Pathology	There is a diffuse, non-necrotizing granulomatous inflammation in the uvea. The choroid is markedly thickened but the choriocapillaris is spared. DFN consist of epithelioid cells between Bruch's membrane and the retinal pigment epithelium (RPE).
Antigens	Possible inciting antigens suggested include; rhodopsin, retinal soluble antigen and interphotoreceptor retinoid binding protein. Uveal melanin does not show immunopathogenic capacity.
Enucleation	Enucleation of the injured eye before the fellow becomes involved is the only prevention. Early enucleation (within two weeks of the injury) may improve the visual prognosis. The literature on the subject supports all efforts to save an eye with any prospect for useful vision.
Treatment	High-dose intravenous steroids during the first few days have been suggested. Alternatively you can start with oral steroids (60 mg per day) and taper slowly. Cyclosporin A (5 mg /kg) is a potent inhibitor of T-cell function and can be used to reduce the dose of steroids required or to help control refractory disease.
Outcome	With appropriate medical therapy, 70 per cent or more of sympathizing eyes will see 6/18 or better. Over 50 per cent may need long-term systemic steroids and may suffer recurrent relapses.

struck with considerable force the sclera may rupture and orbital injuries, such as blow-out fractures, may also be found. In such circumstances, the damage to the globe is usually catastrophic. Subconjunctival and intraocular haemorrhage may well mask the injuries in these cases. Rupture of the sclera tends to occur around the point of insertion of the extraocular muscles causing protrusion of the uveal tissues and loss of the ocular contents.

Treatment is usually symptomatic, conservative and supportive unless a rupture is suspected. In that case the eye will be soft and the vision very poor and surgical exploration is essential.

The impact of blunt trauma can be documented systematically by considering the anatomical structures involved:

(1) Cornea.
(2) Iris.
(3) Ciliary body.
(4) Lens.
(5) Posterior segment injuries.
(6) Optic nerve.
(7) Optic pathway.

For each of these structures, an appropriate management plan is suggested.

(1) CORNEA

Significant trauma will reduce the endothelial cell count, especially in cases associated with ciliary body disinsertion. Small linear cracks in Descemet's membrane can be seen (cf. birth trauma).

Management

Conservative support is usually all that is required. Post-traumatic corneal oedema will usually clear spontaneously.

(2) IRIS

Mild trauma can result in traumatic mydriasis, iritis and small sphincter ruptures. More severe injury can avulse the iris root leading to iridodialysis (Figs 2.3, 2.4 and 2.5). Damage to any part of the iris, but particularly in the area of the major arterial circle, can result in hyphaema.

Hyphaema

Most blood in the anterior chamber will have been resorbed in four to five days (Fig. 2.6). Extensive bleeding or cases of total ('8-ball' after the black pool ball) hyphaema can be more serious. Persistent hyphaema, especially in conjunction with raised intraocular pressure, can lead to corneal staining. Afro-Caribbean patients and those with poor vision (6/60 or less) and raised IOP may be at an increased risk of a secondary bleed, which will worsen the prognosis.

Management

Patients should be warned that because their iris has been damaged that they may have problems with glare and photophobia. Iris trauma may be associated with ciliary

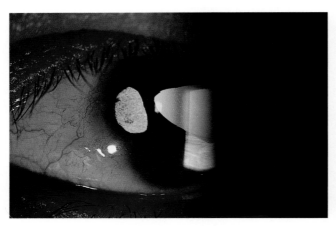

Figure 2.3. Iridodialysis as a result of an injury with a skipping rope.

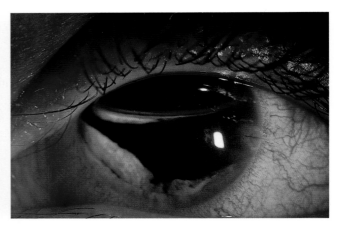

Figure 2.4. Total iridodialysis following severe blunt injury with a thrown bottle. There was an associated giant retinal tear.

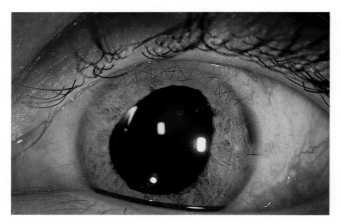

Figure 2.5. The iridodialysis was repaired and a transcleral secondary IOL implanted after vitreo-retinal surgery. A final visual acuity of 6/18 was achieved.

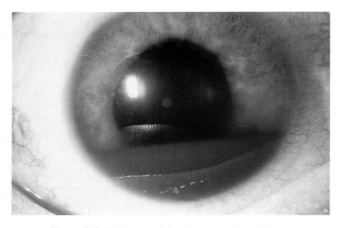

Figure 2.6. Hyphaema following a squash-ball injury.

body disruption so IOP should be monitored regularly. Both glaucoma and hypotony can result. A large iridodialysis will also cause visual problems, especially if it is positioned from 2 to 10 o'clock. The principles of repairing these injuries are described in a series of annotated diagrams (Figs 2.7a–e). The management of hyphaema will depend on the risk of re-bleeding and a suggested protocol is presented in Table 2.6.

(3) CILIARY BODY

Partial ciliary body disinsertion may be caused by blunt trauma. This is seen as 'angle recession' on gonioscopy (Fig. 2.8). You need to carefully examine the fellow eye for signs of a pre-existing primary anomaly. Partial disinsertion appears to compromise aqueous drainage, which may lead to secondary glaucoma (the more clock-hours affected, the greater the risk).

Table 2.6. Hyphaema – treatment depending on the risk of re-bleeding.

Low risk (small bleed, Caucasian)
Outpatient bed rest.
Dilate with g-atropine 1 per cent bd (paralyses the iris and allows posterior segment examination)
Topical prednisolone acetate 0.5 per cent qds

High risk (Afro-Caribbean, raised IOP, secondary bleed, large hyphaema)
In-patient bed rest
Dilate with g-atropine 1 per cent bd
Topical prednisolone acetate 0.5 per cent qds
Medical treatment of IOP (beta-blocker)
Oral antifibrinolytic, e.g. tranexamic acid (25 mg/kg tds)
Oral aminocaproic acid (50 mg/kg, qds) can also be used to help reduce risk of re-bleed.
Consider surgery (washout ± trabeculectomy with 5-fluorouracil if IOP uncontrollable).

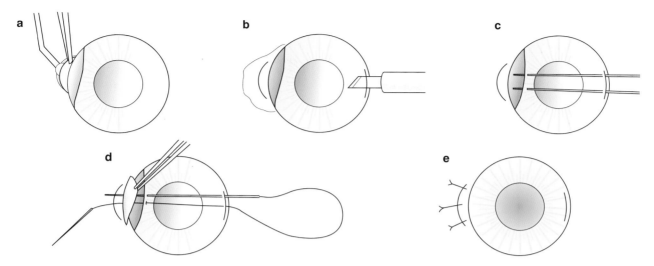

Figure 2.7. Drawings to show the technique of repairing an iris dialysis. (a) A flap of conjunctiva and superficial sclera is lifted in the area of the dialysis. The scleral flap is gently undercut forwards to the limbus using a crescent blade. (b) A counter-incision is made in the cornea on the opposite side of the eye from the dialysis. (c) The AC is filled with Healon®, and using a double-ended suture (long, straight needles, 10-0 Prolene) pass them, one at a time, across the eye and through the disinserted iris root. (d) Push the needles through the angle and out under the scleral flap previously created. Aim to get the tips to emerge further posteriorly than might have at first appeared appropriate. If the needles emerge too far forward, then this gives the effect of hoisting the iris forwards. (e) Pull up the tension on the iris as this is done and when happy that the pupil is central, tie the Prolene threads together. If over-tightened it will be noted that the pupil will be distorted and come to lie eccentrically. If zealous, this suturing can be repeated, giving a broader zone of attachment of the iris periphery. Normally however, a single pair of sutures is all that is needed. Suture the back edge of the scleral flap and close the conjunctiva.

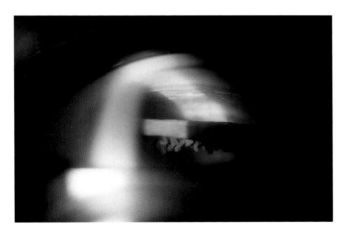

Figure 2.8. Massive angle recession with ciliary body disinsertion causing hypotony.

Management

Ciliary body trauma often leads to a low-grade cyclitis. Consequently, these eyes can often be managed conservatively with topical steroid drops alone. Milder cases should be reviewed regularly for raised IOP. More extensive ciliary body disinsertion may result in hypotony, hence surgical repair (cyclopexy) should be considered. Figure 2.8 is of a patient who had been kicked in his right eye by a horse. Note that the pupil is dilated, the iris limp and the ciliary body hangs on the sagging iris. There is a huge cyclodialysis cleft, which extends far back under the retina. Retinal changes from chronic choroidal effusions were visible.

The surgeon may attempt to close small clefts using argon laser trabeculoplasty or cyclocryotherapy. Surgical repair of the cleft should be considered if it extends for more than two clock-hours or if there is associated macular oedema or choroidal folds with an IOP under 4 mmHg. The technique of cyclopexy is described in Table 2.7 and Fig 2.9.

Table 2.7. Demeler's technique of cyclopexy (see Fig. 2.9).

1. Identify the sector or quadrant of the cyclodialysis cleft.
2. Raise a fornix-based conjuctival flap.
3. Fashion a limbus-based scleral flap. The flap should extend along the full circumference of the cleft (more than one may be needed), be 5 mm wide and reach a depth of 50 per cent of the scleral thickness.
4. The remaining tissue, under the primary scleral flap, should now be opened to create a fornix-based deep scleral flap, which will reveal the ciliary body underneath.
5. A double-ended 10-0 Prolene suture with atraumatic needles is passed through the superficial tissues of the ciliary body, and then the needles are pushed through the deep flap and tied. The knots will be buried on the deep surface of the superficial flap.
6. The superficial flap is securely closed with multiple 10-0 nylon sutures (cf. a trabeculectomy where some leakage through the flap is required). This buries the Prolene suture ends.
7. The conjunctiva is closed with 10-0 nylon.

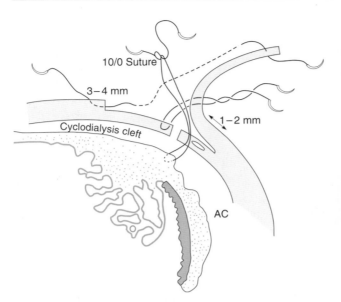

Figure 2.9. Demeler's technique of cyclopexy.

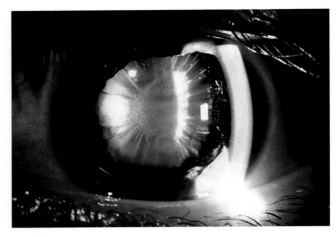

Figure 2.11. Crenellations of the capsule with 360 degrees of zonular damage and marked phacodenesis.

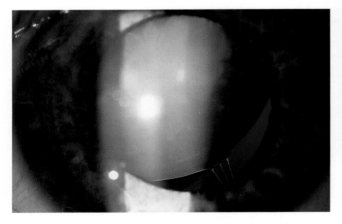

Figure 2.10. Lens subluxation showing remaining zonular fibres.

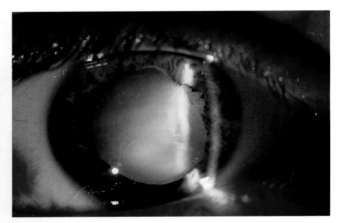

Figure 2.12. Capsule and sphincter rupture with a traumatic cataract.

(4) LENS

The force of ocular compression is transmitted to the iris, which in turn can lead the iris to impact on the lens, leaving a pigment ring on the anterior capsule. Severe damage may partially (Fig. 2.10) or completely dislocate the crystalline lens. Subluxation may be seen as irido- or phacodenesis and may present as crenellations of the capsule (Fig. 2.11). The traumatized lens may become cataractous, especially if there is a breach of the anterior capsule (Fig. 2.12). Vitreous may be forced into the anterior chamber in a phakic or pseudophakic eye. In these cases it is squeezed through the zonular gaps by the increased posterior segment pressure.

Management

The patient with simple phacodenesis should be warned that cataract or glaucoma might develop in the future. If the displacement is such that the visual axis is rendered effectively aphakic, a contact lens can be tried to correct the vision. If the vision is unsatisfactory and confused because of the intrusion of the lens edge into the pupil, the lens can be surgically removed. Anterior dislocation requires urgent surgical attention, as there is a risk of angle closure glaucoma.

Lens surgery in the presence of zonular damage requires specialized techniques. In milder cases the introduction of a capsular tension ring into the capsular fornix may allow removal of the lens with phacoemulsification and capsular implantation of the IOL.

In more advanced subluxation, intracapsular extraction may be the only realistic option. However, new variations on the design of capsular tension rings designed by Dr Robert J Cionni (with extra tails and eyes) make it possible to suture the ring to the iris or sclera before commencing lens surgery (Fig. 2.13). The lens is thus stabilized, and if the lens is reasonably soft it can be removed with phaco and an IOL implanted. If the patient is elderly, such ocular gymnastics will be impossible because of the hardness of nucleus, and it is prudent then to merely remove the lens and consider a sutured, possibly secondary IOL implantation.

(5) POSTERIOR SEGMENT INJURIES

There are three mechanisms by which an object can cause blunt damage in the posterior segment:

(a) Direct injury.

(b) Indirect (contre-coup) injury.

(c) Antero-posterior compression.

(a) Direct injury

A projectile which ricochets off the eye, instead of perforating it, can lead to sclopetaria (traumatic chorioretinal rupture). The damage sustained is usually anterior to the equator. An area of retina, retinal pigment epithelium and choroid retracts to reveal the sclera (Fig. 2.14). Intragel or pre-retinal haemorrhage can obscure the signs. The risk of secondary retinal detachment is low but long-term follow-up is advised.

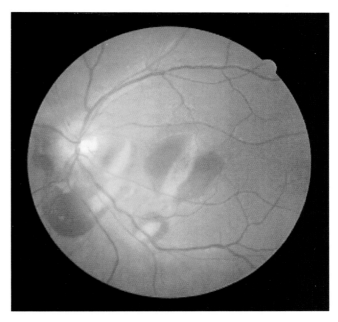

Figure 2.14. Traumatic chorioretinal rupture (sclopetaria).

(b) Contre-coup injuries

These lesions are seen within tissues opposite to the site of impact. In this way an object hitting the cornea will lead to problems in the macular region that may include commotio retinae, choroidal rupture or a traumatic macular hole. Retinal detachments can also result but these are more common with anteroposterior compression injuries.

Commotio retinae is characterized by a whitening of the retina, which represents deep retinal oedema. This retinal contusion looks similar to the oedema and ischaemia following an artery occlusion (Fig. 2.15). If it involves the macula, the fovea is often spared giving the appearance of a (pseudo) cherry-red spot. The oedema usually settles

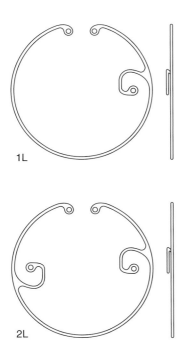

Figure 2.13. Innovative capsular tension ring designs (courtesy of John Weiss).

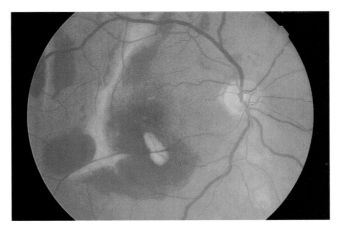

Figure 2.15. Retinal commotio.

in a few days and vision usually returns to normal. Extensive commotio affecting the posterior pole may lead to permanent visual loss.

Purtscher's retinopathy, caused by multiple small emboli following severe head trauma, can resemble commotio. One or both eyes may be affected with posterior pole retinal ischaemia with associated retinal haemorrhages (Fig. 2.16). Vision may recover but there is no treatment.

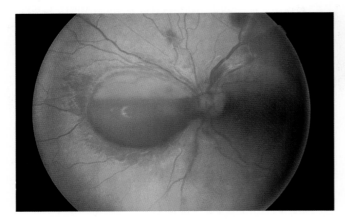

Figure 2.16. Purtscher's retinopathy; there is a subhyaloid haemorrhage as well as retinal haemorrhages following a seat belt injury.

A choroidal rupture will be commonly seen as a white crescent-like concentric break near the optic disc. It represents a breach of the choroid, retinal pigment epithelium and Bruch's membrane. Initially, the lesion is often covered by pre-retinal haem. If the rupture or the overlying blood affects the macula, vision will be affected. As the blood clears, the curvilinear scar will become visible and there may be some pigmentary discolouration. As Bruch's membrane has been breached, there is a risk of secondary neovascularization through the scar. This will present as visual distortion (e.g. on an Amsler chart) if the macula is involved and will need investigation with fluorescein angiography. More peripheral neovascular membranes may only present once they have bled into the vitreous.

Macular holes complicate around 1 in 20 cases of blunt trauma. They are caused by the rapid avulsion of the vitreous at the macula leading to a focal distraction of retinal tissue (Fig. 2.17). A traumatic macular hole looks very similar in size and shape to an idiopathic age-related lesion and leads to the same central scotoma. Surgery for traumatic macular holes is currently being evaluated.

(c) Antero-posterior compression injuries

As an object hits the eye along its visual axis, the cornea will be pushed towards the macula. This will rapidly increase the equatorial diameter, which can lead to vitreous base avulsion, retinal dialysis, retinal detachment and giant retinal tears.

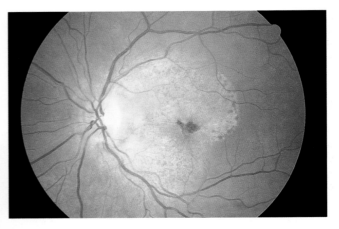

Figure 2.17. Traumatic macular hole with surrounding chorio-retinal atrophy.

Vitreous base avulsion may or may not be associated with a traumatic retinal detachment. It is seen as an arcuate band overlying the peripheral retina (with its convexity pointing at the macula). Vitreous base avulsion should be treated with cryotherapy or photocoagulation to the surrounding intact base. This can reduce the risk of retinal complications due to vitreous traction.

Retinal dialysis is where the retina has separated from the pars plana epithelium at the ora serrata. It is seen as a slit at the ora, which gapes on scleral indentation (Fig. 2.18). There may be an associated retinal detachment but this is often localized, especially in infero-temporal dialyses, which are more common. The treatment is laser or cryotherapy retinopexy to prevent the extension of any detachment. Where there is pre-existing subretinal fluid, scleral buckling is advisable.

Trauma can lead to holes anywhere in the retina. Horseshoe-shaped tears, especially those with vitreous traction, are at high risk of progressing to retinal detachment. If there are areas of abnormal vitreo-retinal adhesion

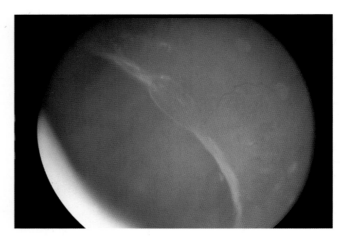

Figure 2.18. Retinal dialysis.

e.g. lattice degeneration, these will often be the weakest zones, most liable to damage. Depending on their position, flat holes can be treated with laser or cryotherapy retinopexy. Detachments may require external or internal surgical repair, the details of which are beyond this volume.

Giant retinal tears occur at the interface between the posterior edge of the vitreous base and the retina. They are circumferential breaks that extend for three or more clock-hours (Fig. 2.19). Scleral buckling is rarely successful and the usual surgical treatment is a pars planar vitrectomy with gas or silicone oil exchange. These operations, especially if delayed, are often complicated by the development of proliferative vitreo-retinopathy.

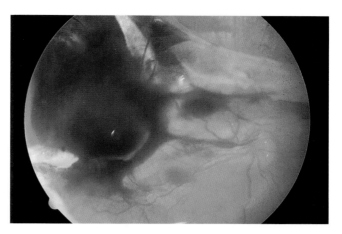

Figure 2.20. Fundal appearance after optic nerve avulsion.

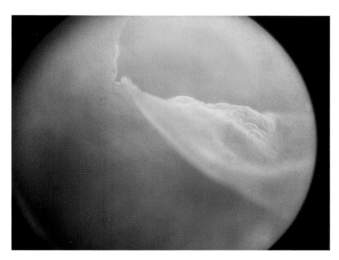

Figure 2.19. Giant retinal tear.

OPTIC NERVE

The optic nerve may be damaged in two ways:

(a) Direct injury, e.g. avulsion or mechanical transection/compression.

(b) Indirect injury via its blood supply (vasa nervorum).

(a) Direct injury

Avulsion or anterior transection leads to a characteristic fundal picture of haemorrhage and infarction (Fig. 2.20) as the ophthalmic artery is involved. More posterior damage may be unrecognizable on fundoscopy at its acute presentation but will eventually lead to optic atrophy.

Intraorbital bleeding, especially if within the muscle cone, can rapidly lead to compressive optic neuropathy. Performing a lateral cantholysis and canthotomy can instantly relieve the pressure from a retrobulbar haemorrhage (Figs 2.21a and b).

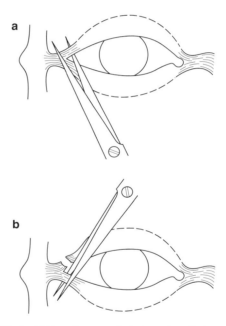

Figure 2.21. (a, b) Emergency cantholysis and canthotomy – both superior and inferior limbs of the lateral canthal tendon are cut with sharp-pointed scissors.

(b) Indirect injury

Damage to the optic nerve canal may disrupt the optic nerve's blood supply, the vasa nervorum. This can lead to a 'silent' optic neuropathy that is not recognizable on magnetic resonance imaging (MRI). Rarely, the vasa can rupture and lead to bleeding within the optic nerve sheath. This can lead to the clinical appearance of a central retinal vein occlusion. Imaging will reveal enlargement of the optic nerve sheath, which can occasionally be treated with an expeditious optic nerve sheath fenestration. High-dose intravenous corticosteroids may reduce lipid peroxidation and may limit the damage (30 mg/kg of methylprednisolone over a 30 min period). Further pulses of methylprednisolone should be given over the first 48 hours and subsequently oral steroids should be given on a tapering dose. It should be used within 8 hours of the initial injury for maximal effect. Extracranial optic canal decompression can be considered if medical treatment fails.

OPTIC PATHWAY

Whilst traumatic optic neuropathy is well recognized, you should remember that facial and cervico-cranial injuries can cause chiasm and occipital cortex damage that may also compromise vision.

Chiasmal trauma should be suspected where there has been frontal and basilar skull fractures. Neuro-ophthalmic sequelae include bitemporal hemianopia, diabetes insipidus and hypopituitarism. Traumatic carotid aneurysms, carotid cavernous fistulae and cerebrospinal fluid leaks may also occur. Bilateral afferent pathway damage will lead to light-near dissociation with pupillary constriction present with accommodation alone. MRI is the modality of choice to identify the site of injury. Optic atrophy will eventually develop which can be seen on fundoscopy. Early liaison with neurosurgical colleagues is essential. High-dose intravenous corticosteroids may be beneficial.

With normal fundoscopy, bilateral visual loss with normal pupil reactions suggests occipital cortex damage. Injury may result from a direct blow or from hypoperfusion secondary to vascular compression or systemic hypotension. Patients with occipital tip dysfunction will present with bilateral, congruent central scotomata, which can resolve with time. Injury to the occipital cortex results in symmetrical homonymous visual field defects that spare central fixation. MRI is very useful in delineating the area of damage.

PERFORATING INJURIES

Sharp injuries vary in their extent and depth, and retained foreign bodies must always be suspected. Entry wounds can be minute and yet sufficient for the penetration of the missile into the posterior segment. The history should alert to the possibility that a fragment may have entered the eye, e.g. following an explosion. After any penetrating injury, appropriate radiological investigations (X-ray, CT scan, not MRI,) must always be done to exclude an intraocular foreign body (IOFB).

Simple wounds, such as a corneal laceration, should have excellent visual recovery if accurately repaired. It is reasonable to argue in such cases that the primary surgery should only be done by the most skilled medical staff, since the quality of that repair will affect the functional profile of the cornea. In contrast, the grossly injured eye may be repaired by a more junior doctor (with adequate supervision if required) because visual returns from the repair are likely to be limited, no matter how well the eye is repaired. However, no eye should ever be written off as a training exercise and appropriate support must always be available.

Intraocular foreign body (IOFB)

An IOFB should be ruled out after any perforating injury. Even in the absence of a suggestive history of contact with a fast-moving projectile, an IOFB must be deliberately excluded. IOFBs may be single or multiple, or may fragment. The momentum of a large IOFB will cause severe disruption, much more than a small or sharp projectile. A fast-moving, sharp foreign body can leave next-to-no scar through an upper lid but can cause catastrophic intraocular damage.

As a foreign body enters the eye, it may become embedded anywhere, in the cornea, anterior or posterior chamber, the lens or the posterior segment. In the posterior segment, the IOFB may lie in or on the retina. Here it will be wrapped in blood and vitreous, possibly hiding a retinal perforation and contusion (see Fig. 2.22). Other damage occurs as it ricochets within the eye. It may transfix the sclera or doubly penetrate, coming to rest in the orbit.

Identifying any IOFB is crucial to avoid the disastrous damage, which can occur when salts and radicals are released from retained metallic fragments, e.g. chalcosis and siderosis. The medico-legal consequences of failing to suspect, diagnose, image and remove an IOFB are well rehearsed (see Figs 2.23–2.26).

Surgical principles

Perforation of the globe should be considered a relative medical emergency. Removal of any foreign material and necrotic tissue, and the prompt closure of the wound, if

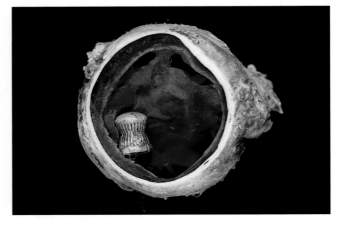

Figure 2.22. Retained air gun pellet lying in the vitreous in an enucleated eye, with massive disruption of the retina and ocular contents.

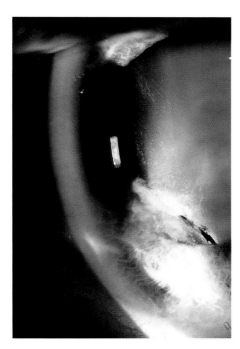

Figure 2.23. Peripheral corneal, iris and lens perforation from a minute foreign body.

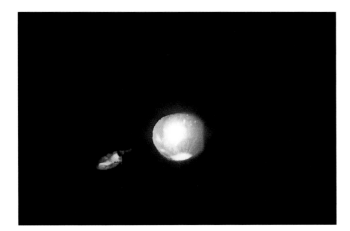

Figure 2.24. The same patient showing the red reflex through the iris perforation.

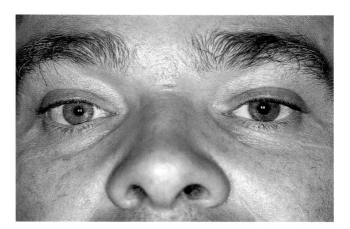

Figure 2.25. Heterochromia in a patient with siderosis bulbi.

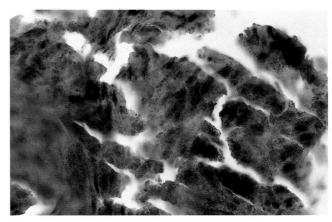

Figure 2.26. Haematoxylin and eosin staining of disintegrating foreign body and retina specimen taken from peripheral retina of the patient in Fig. 2.25.

required, will reduce the risks of post-traumatic endophthalmitis and improve the eye's prognosis. Primary repair should be performed as soon as possible but within 24 hours at the most.

The surgical goals when attempting primary repair of any traumatic injury should respect and reflect the need to restore global integrity, maintain optically clear, non-astigmatic central visual axis and to conserve all viable tissue. Primary repair may be the only surgery required, e.g. in a simple peripheral corneal laceration. With more advanced, complex injuries, primary repair may be performed to restore globe integrity in the hope of some ocular

salvage, with the surgeon planning to do a definitive procedure at a later time.

The principles of the approach to a perforating injury of the eye are:

(1) Identify the full extent of the wound itself.
(2) Identify which ocular tissues have been involved/ lost.
(3) Conserve as much viable tissue as possible (see also Table 2.8).
(4) Ensure water-tight closure.
(5) Plan appropriate reconstruction.

(1) THE EXTENT OF THE WOUND

Sharp perforating injuries fall all into two groups. First, those involving unidirectional, radial perforation with a sharp pointed object, such as a needle, dart (Fig. 2.27) or yucca leaf. The external entry site may self-seal and appear

Table 2.8. General rules for managing prolapsed tissue at primary repair.

- Abscise anything that has been extruded any distance, e.g. onto cheek
- Shiny, pigmented tissue remote from the wound edge should be excised with long-bladed scissors up to the wound edge
- Prolapsing vitreous should be abscised up to the level of the wound. This may require tidying up with a vitreous cutter.
- Pigmented tissue traversing the wound, i.e. retina or iris, should be handled gently and, if possible, reposited back into the eye
- Most tissue will lose its viability if it has been out of the eye for more than 24 hours.

innocuous although many tissues, including cornea, iris, lens and even retina may have been damaged. Additional movements of the injuring instrument will extend the wound (Fig. 2.28) and cause much greater damage than a simple 'in and out' stab. This type of perforation commonly causes a gaping wound, and loss of the ocular contents is readily apparent. Surgery is the first line of management.

The extent of any globe rupture must be visualized. With forceful blunt trauma, corneo-scleral ruptures may spiral

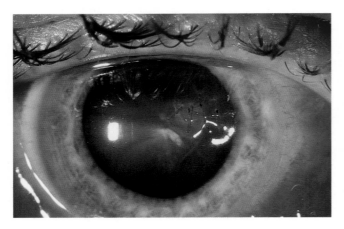

Figure 2.27. Corneal and lens damage from a dart injury.

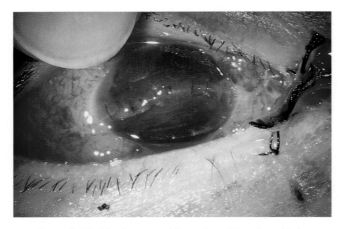

Figure 2.28. Massive corneal laceration with a sharp blade.

posteriorly requiring extensive conjunctival recession in order to gauge the trauma extent. Occasionally, the recti muscles may have to be disinserted. The use of a standard eyelid speculum for this type of surgery will squeeze the eye, risking further tissue prolapse. It is better to use an independent eyelid speculum, which can be distracted without increasing intraocular pressure.

(2) IDENTIFYING THE TISSUES THAT ARE INVOLVED OR LOST

A methodical examination of the eye, both pre- and per-operatively will help you to plan the primary and secondary repair. The position, size and shape of the outer wound, whether through cornea or sclera, will have prognostic implications regarding visual potential. The deeper the injuries, the more complex the damage will be and the repair needs to be more involved.

Cornea/sclera

There are five categories of traumatic wounds:

  (a) Small, simple corneal.
  (b) Large, simple corneal.
  (c) Complex corneal.
  (d) Corneo-limbal.
  (e) Scleral/mid-segment.

(a) Small simple corneal wounds

Sharp objects such as pieces of glass or a knife generally cause these injuries. Provided there is no rotational or tangential movement, the wound is usually a linear laceration without contusion. There is no tissue loss and the wound is regular (Figs 2.29 and 2.30). There may be no shallowing or leakage in the anterior chamber (confirmed by doing a Seidel test, with 2 per cent fluorescein). The wound may be shelved or oblique allowing a degree of self-sealing.

In patients, such as children or the mentally handicapped, because of the risk of the patient further injuring the eye it is safer to place sutures in these small wounds.

(b) Large, simple corneal wounds

There are more extensive lesions, which obviously need suturing (Figs 2.31 and 2.32). Here, there is significant shallowing of the anterior chamber, which may be associated with an iris knuckle to the wound. There is a significant risk of infection and/or prolapse of ocular contents with the possibility of incarceration.

(c) Complex corneal injuries

Damage with a blunt object often leads to a larger stellate corneal wound with tissue loss or maceration (Fig. 2.33). The wound edge is often severely irregular, with marked implications regarding corneal astigmatism following primary repair (Fig. 2.34a–c).

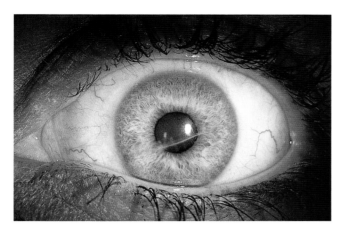

Figure 2.29. Clean, small corneal laceration.

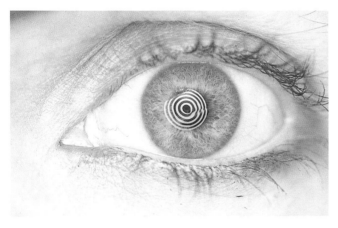

Figure 2.30. Keratoscopic picture of the same patient showing irregularity of the rings following injury.

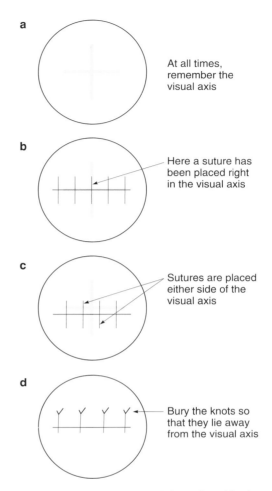

a

At all times, remember the visual axis

b

Here a suture has been placed right in the visual axis

c

Sutures are placed either side of the visual axis

d

Bury the knots so that they lie away from the visual axis

Figure 2.32. Drawings to show the technique of repairing large simple corneal lacerations.

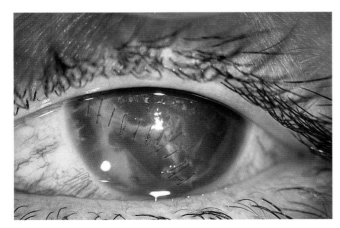

Figure 2.31. Post-operative view after repair of a Y-shaped corneal wound.

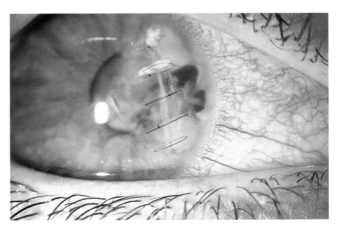

Figure 2.33. Here, a peripheral corneal injury has resulted in loss of tissue making it difficult to close the wound without gross distortion. Further surgery will be required.

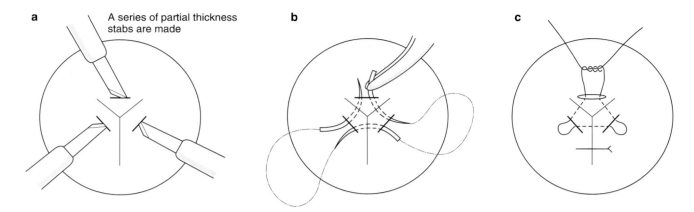

a A series of partial thickness stabs are made

b

c

Figure 2.34. Drawings to show the technique of repairing complex corneal wound (Eisner's method). (a) Make a series of partial-thickness stabs between the limbs of the laceration. (b) Suture with 10-0 nylon, passing the needle across the laceration from the depths of the stab wounds making a clover-leaf purse-string suture. (c) The knot is tied to lie in the depths of the wound. A corneal graft is usually later required.

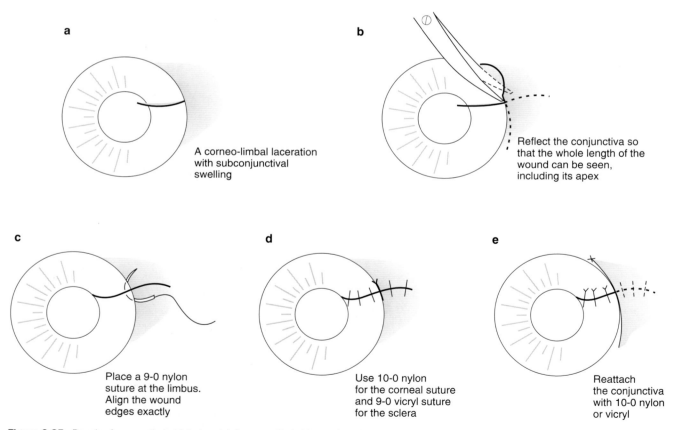

a A corneo-limbal laceration with subconjunctival swelling

b Reflect the conjunctiva so that the whole length of the wound can be seen, including its apex

c Place a 9-0 nylon suture at the limbus. Align the wound edges exactly

d Use 10-0 nylon for the corneal suture and 9-0 vicryl suture for the sclera

e Reattach the conjunctiva with 10-0 nylon or vicryl

Figure 2.35. Repair of corneo-limbal injuries. (a) A corneo-limbal laceration with subconjunctival swelling. (b) Reflect the conjunctiva so that the whole length of the wound can be seen. (c) Place a single 9-0 nylon suture at the limbus to align the wound edges exactly. (d) Use 10-0 nylon for the corneal sutures and 9-0 vicryl to close the scleral wound. (e) Reattach the conjunctiva with 10-0 nylon or vicryl. Bury the corneal knots. If it proves impossible to bury the 9-0 nylon at the limbus, replace this with a 10-0 nylon mattress suture.

Chapter 3

History and examination

INTRODUCTION

With complicated surgery, or complex injuries, the visual potential depends on the extent of the damage especially with regard to glaucoma, retinal, macular or optic nerve problems. Time spent taking a detailed history and performing a thorough examination will enable you to formulate a therapeutic plan that is appropriate to the patient.

HISTORY

A full general and ophthalmic history is required. Because both external trauma and complicated primary surgery may have litigious connotations, it is important to pay close attention to the details of the patient's story. This may be invaluable later.

Your clinical record should be clearly dated and should note who, if anyone, accompanied the patient to your consultation. Establishing the patient's occupation and their marital status helps to start conversations and may be important later.

The salient incident

The patient may have had previous complicated primary surgery under your care or someone else's. Their account of the chronology of events including medical and surgical treatments offered and performed will help you to gauge their perception of their management thus far. The names of the people and third parties concerned should be recorded.

Details of any traumatic event should be taken in a similar way. Paying careful attention to the fine points of the history will help later if you are required to produce a witness statement.

Current symptoms

The 'salient incident' may be a cascade of events ending in the patient's current situation. They may be suffering from discomfort, irritation or pain. The nature of these may indicate their underlying cause, e.g. loose corneal sutures may lead to a sharp pain, whereas low-grade grumbling uveitis will cause a deeper ache that is worsened in light or by trying to read. Vision may have been affected. Knowing the status of the eye(s) before the incident will allow you to estimate its impact on sight. Vision may have been affected immediately or may have gradually deteriorated over time. Double vision may not have been reported previously but the history of a manifest or latent squint may suggest decompensation. Ghosting and frank diplopia are clearly different symptoms with different aetiologies. A subluxated IOL can lead to optical aberrations which may be chromatic, spherical or prismatic.

The patient may be complaining of systemic problems such as dizziness, headaches and nausea. All or none of these can be related to ocular pathology.

Main problem

Whilst the patient may have a string of complaints or symptoms, it is useful for him/her and you to single out the main concern. This may be visual function, reduced acuity or diplopia, discomfort and/or pain or cosmetic appearance (due to a squint or corneal scarring, for example).

Perceived dysfunction

The incident may have led to the patient having to take time off work or to have problems self-caring. As importantly, in some cases, leisure pursuits may have had to be stopped. Self-esteem or confidence may have been affected resulting in psychosocial problems and introversion.

Past ocular history

Previous injuries or operations should be carefully documented. Details from any previous hospital visits can be helpful in filling in the missing pieces of the story. Pre-existing problems, such as amblyopia, macular degeneration or diabetic retinopathy, may lead to the patient ascribing too much blame on to the salient incident. They may also preclude a satisfactory visual outcome from your proposed reconstruction.

Past medical history

The patient's general health may have suffered as a result of the original 'injury'. A traumatic accident may have damaged non-ocular structures leading to physical disability. The initial incident, or the medical treatment during or following it, may have caused psychological damage. The patient may be depressed and may be on medication. He/she may be angry and contemplating legal action. The patient's mind-set may be such that further surgery may not be an option in the short term. Psychiatric problems or mental incapacity may make a patient more likely to rub the eye after surgery. This may obviously compromise the final outcome.

Treatment

Aside from any surgery that may have already been done, it is important to record a drug history which will include any topical medication the patient has used or is currently using.

Some systemic medications may affect the choice of further surgery, e.g. warfarin, which may complicate local anaesthesia.

Patient expectations

It is worth clearly stating in the records what the patient's goals are for further surgery and whether these match your own. They may have very unreal expectations, hence pre-operative counselling is crucial.

EXAMINATION

The examination of any eye considered for reconstructive surgery should begin with an assessment of visual ability, the current situation, and visual potential, which will describe the realistic prognosis for vision post-operatively.

During the systematic examination of the eye, a special note should be made of pathological processes that are 'active' and which may lead to a deterioration and which may be symptomatic (redness, pain, photophobia etc.). 'Static' pathology, such as scars and membranes, reflect the history of insults to the eye but are non-progressive problems.

During the consultation, you should be asking yourself the following questions:

(1) What needs to be done?
(2) How can it be done?

(3) What else will help in planning a therapeutic approach?
(4) What is a realistic plan?

Such a problem-based examination will concentrate on the surgical pathology present and identify that which threatens to cause future problems.

Vision

Visual acuity should be measured and recorded using a Logmar or Snellen chart. The use of a pin-hole will overcome mild-to-moderate refractive errors and some corneal distortion. If aphakic, a +10.00 dioptre lens should be used with a pin-hole to obtain a meaningful acuity. From a recent audit, 80 per cent of reconstructive surgeries were performed to improve vision, 15 per cent to improve symptoms of discomfort and 5 per cent to address a cosmetic problem.

Visual potential describes the best guess of the function a patient can expect post-operatively assuming surgery goes well (Table 3.1). A history of long-term visual impairment or amblyopia may limit post-operative visual gains. Clearly, if the major impediment to vision is media opacity, and this is removed, the visual outcome will be good. If, however, there is optic nerve or macular pathology, clearing the visual axis may have little functional benefit. If it is felt that the visual potential is poor, the arguments and justification to proceed to tectonic surgery must be given a different emphasis to those where there is good potential for vision.

Table 3.1. Causes of visual loss in eyes coming for reconstruction.

Anterior segment	cornea	astigmatism, scar, oedema
	anterior chamber	pupillary membrane (occlusio pupillae)
		blood clot
		cyclitic membrane
Mid-segment	lens	aphakia, subluxation, cataract
		complicated psuedophakos
		errors of lens power
Posterior segment	vitreous	vitreous haemorrhage, vitirits
	retina	cystoid macular oedema detachment, toxic (secondary to IOFB)
		macular hole/scar
		choroidal tear
	optic nerve	transection, contusion, toxic damage, glaucomatous damage (secondary raised IOP)

Assessment of visual potential

PUPIL REACTIONS

Direct and consensual reactions will indicate the integrity of the afferent and efferent pathways to the iris in each eye. Even if the iris in the damaged eye cannot be utilized, performing the 'swinging flashlight test' whilst looking at the healthy eye will be sufficient. If neither iris is functional, a subjective measure, asking the patient to grade the brightness of your light from 0 to 10 ('brightness appreciation test'), can indicate relative dysfunction.

PROJECTION OF LIGHT

If vision is poor, counting fingers or less, and if there are dense medial opacities, the integrity of the retinal quadrants can be judged by asking the patient to say from which direction the light is being shone.

VISUAL FIELDS

With central opacities, visual acuity may be poor. Testing a patient's peripheral field can help to demonstrate an intact optic nerve. Where a previous insult has caused secondary glaucoma, perimetry may be important in terms of prognosis as well as pre- and post-operative treatment.

ELECTROPHYSIOLOGY

Visual-evoked potentials and electroretinography are useful to objectively assess the health of the optic nerve and retina, especially in cases of possible retinal toxicity associated with an IOFB.

Surgical anatomy

This part of the examination should be directed at identifying and distinguishing what 'should' be done and what 'could' be done. One or more surgical steps may be needed to sort out the problems, and the therapeutic possibilities will be determined by the pathology encountered. By the same token, this part of the examination should also identify what cannot be expected for any given eye. Some structural problems and nervous damage will preclude a good visual outcome. The possibility of surgical and post-operative complications may be suggested by the clinical findings.

You should ask yourself the following as you run through a systematic ocular examination:

(1) Is there any active pathology?
(2) Which membranes and/or tissues will need cleaning/replacing?
(3) What is available to reconstruct the pupil?
(4) How and where will an IOL be implanted?
(5) What structural problems will preclude a good visual outcome?
(6) What complications are to be expected?

The final aim of treatment is a permanent improvement in the appearance, comfort and function of the eye. The patient will want to know for what sort of therapeutic contract or plan they will be 'signing-up' to.

ACTIVE PATHOLOGY

Patients with active pathology present with symptoms of pain and discomfort or tenderness. The consistency of the symptoms can lead to social problems, emotional distress and loss of employment. The progressive nature of these pathological changes threatens determination in the clinical situation. Where such active pathology is present, medical or surgical intervention is indicated to prevent deterioration. Examples of such active pathology are presented in Table 3.2 and in Figs 3.1–3.17.

Anterior uveitis is usually symptomatic from whatever cause. Low-grade iris irritation, from a vitreous tag or oversized anterior chamber IOL, can lead to cells and flare in the anterior chamber. Evidence of previous inflammation can be seen as anterior or posterior synechiae or pupillary membranes. The mere presence of a significant amount of inflammatory debris in the anterior chamber may suggest that an irritating problem remains and needs treatment. In contrast, patients with historical damage and long-standing problems such as corneal scars, have non-progressive problems. Whilst this type of pathology may interfere with vision, the eye itself is usually pain-free and there is rarely a risk of continuing deterioration. In these situations, surgical intervention is optional (see Table 3.3).

Table 3.2. Active pathology.

- Proud sutures (giant papillary changes on the tarsal conjunctiva)
- Anterior uveitis (ciliary flush, cells, flare)
- Corneal oedema or infiltration
- Neovascularization (pannus, corneal scars)
- Distorted pupils due to vitreous incarceration and anterior chamber inflammation
- Vitreous traction (antero-posterior and transgel to the vitreous base)
- Complicated pseudophakia (unstable or malpositioned IOL, cellular deposits)
- Glaucoma or hypotony

Table 3.3. Static pathology.

Corneal scars/opacities
Damaged or incomplete iris
Cyclitic membranes or capsular scars
Reduced vision (see Table 3.1)

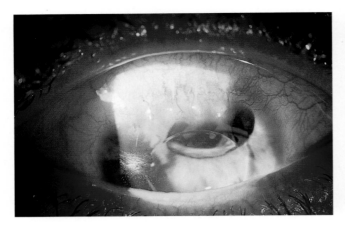

Figure 3.1. Sutures with proud ends.

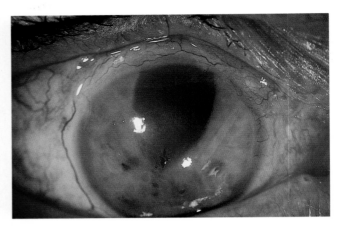

Figure 3.4. Corneal oedema following complicated cataract extraction.

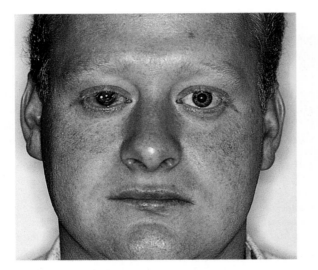

Figure 3.2. Intensely inflamed right eye following complicated anterior chamber (AC) implant.

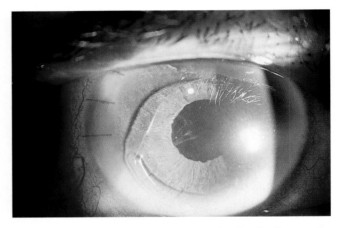

Figure 3.5. The AC IOL has sunk in the anterior chamber because it was too short.

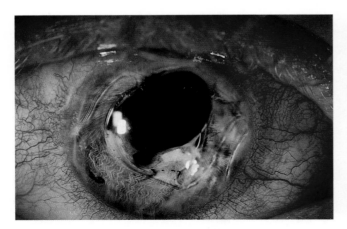

Figure 3.3. Close up of Fig. 3.2 showing AC IOL with incarcerated vitreous and capsule. Glaucoma and cystoid macular oedema prevented full visual return after reconstruction.

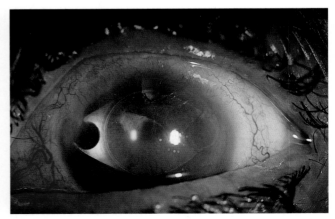

Figure 3.6. Worst 'lobster-claw' AC lens with an intense uveitis.

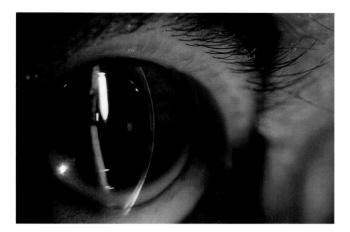

Figure 3.7. The AC IOL has been implanted back to front. This is demonstrated dramatically by the slit of the microscope.

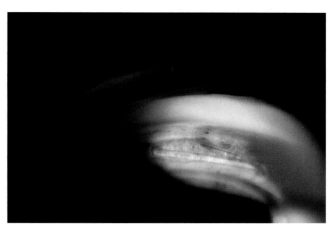

Figure 3.10. Gonioscopy of the same patient as Fig. 3.9 showing adhesions around the haptics.

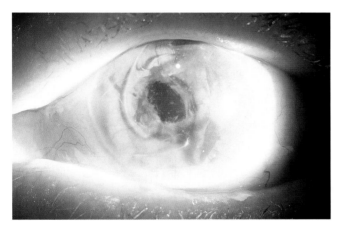

Figure 3.8. Active bleeding in the anterior chamber after implantation of an AC IOL in a patient with rubeosis.

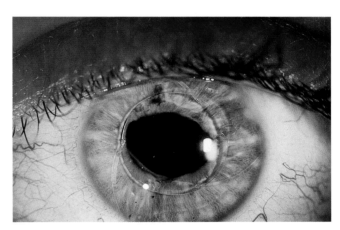

Figure 3.11. Three-legged AC IOL (Dubroff) causing chronic headache. The patient had undergone a craniotomy to try and find the cause of her headache.

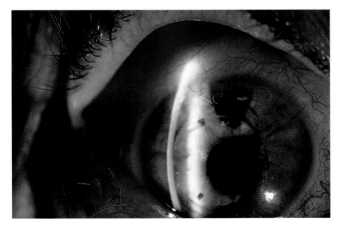

Figure 3.9. An intensely inflamed eye, with cystoid macular oedema. This patient has an AC closed-loop IOL with aggressive angle 'zip-up'.

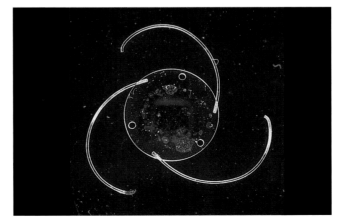

Figure 3.12. The explanted Dubroff lens.

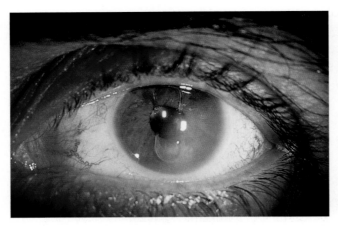

Figure 3.13. Binkhorst iridocapsular lens implanted back to front (note the loops causing corneal decompensation and oedema).

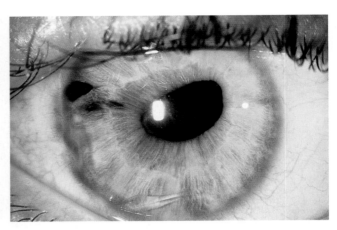

Figure 3.16. A glass foreign body was found in the anterior chamber of this patient who presented for reconstructive surgery (please insert arrow to point to the glass IOFB). If the glass had been left, corneal decompensation would have occurred (see also Fig. 3.18).

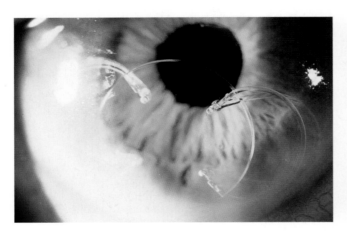

Figure 3.14. Binkhorst lens which has dislocated into the anterior chamber.

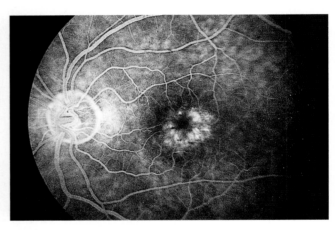

Figure 3.17. Flourescein angiogram showing the petaloid appearance of cystoid macular oedema.

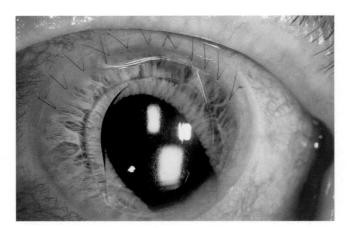

Figure 3.15. As this AC IOL was implanted into the eye, the lower haptic caught vitreous and iris.

MEDIA OPACITIES

Corneal opacity will only hamper vision if it affects the visual axis. Peripheral scars may, however, lead to astigmatism, which becomes less regular the nearer to the visual axis it is. Central corneal pathology may be due to lipid deposition from a neovascular tuft or from a previous perforating injury. In the latter there may be adhesion of internal ocular tissues to the corneal wound, e.g. iris or vitreous. Diffuse corneal opacity can result from endothelial decompensation, or from limbal stem cell failure, resulting in transdifferentiation of the corneal epithelium. Repetitive endothelial trauma, from a foreign body or unstable IOL in the anterior chamber, can also lead to corneal decompensation.

If peripheral, the opacity can often be ignored. If central, but localized, a rotational autograft can be performed.

Where there is extensive corneal decompensation, the only recourse may be a penetrating keratoplasty (Fig. 3.18).

Corneal astigmatism may result from previous surgical wounds. Where there has been previous wound collapse, there may be marked against-the-rule astigmatism which may require a wedge excision for correction (see Fig. 3.19).

The patient may have a traumatic cataract. This may be focal or diffuse. The crystalline lens may be unstable, due to traumatic zonular dehiscence or an inherited weakness such as Marfan's (Fig. 3.20), resulting in phaco- or irido-donesis. The patient may have been rendered aphakic by an injury or a previous operation. The latter may have been

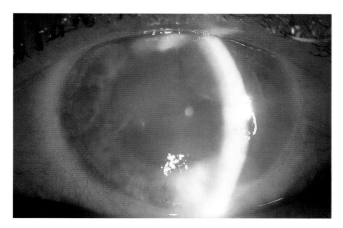

Figure 3.18. Corneal decompensation secondary to a glass IOFB.

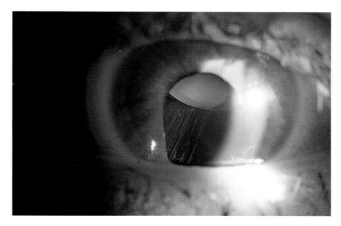

Figure 3.20. Superiorly dislocated Marfan's lens seen through optical iridectomy. Retinal examination revealed a detachment.

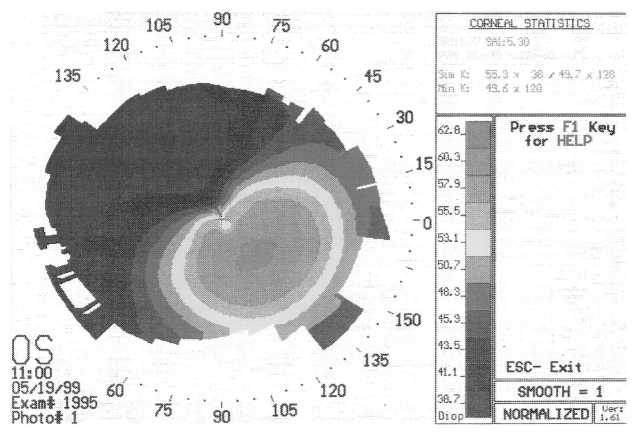

Figure 3.19. Corneal topography of collapsed wound.

an intracapsular procedure, where no capsular remnant would be expected, or extracapsular where residua of the capsule may be present.

If pseudophakic, the patient may have a decentred or unstable IOL. This could lead to significant spherical aberration if the peripheral optic is in the visual axis. If displaced inferiorly, the IOL will show the typical 'sunset' sign (Fig. 3.21).

Vitreous haemorrhage or inflammatory debris may also cause media opacity and should be included in any differential list.

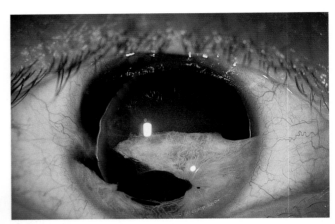

Figure 3.22. Traumatic partial aniridia.

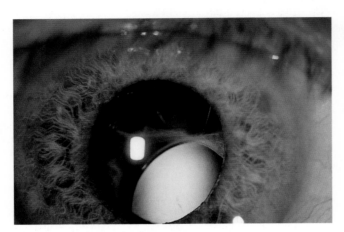

Figure 3.21. 'Sunset sign' of an inferiorly displaced IOL.

IDENTIFYING STRUCTURES FOR IRIS AND PUPILLARY RECONSTRUCTION

Damaged iris, tethered by previous wound involvement or inflammation, may itself block the visual axis. More commonly, there has been tissue loss at the time of trauma, which will lead to a problem with glare unless dealt with appropriately. There may be a complete absence of iris tissue or only partial loss (Fig. 3.22). The existing iris may be adherent to lens or capsule (posterior synechiae) or to the cornea (anterior synechiae). The pupil may be completely occluded by an inflammatory membrane.

The remaining iris should be considered in the following terms:

(1) Is there sufficient tissue to support an iris-sutured IOL if required?

(2) Is there sufficient tissue to re-fashion an adequate pupil?

(3) If the answer to question 2 is no, should an artificial pupil system be considered?

The answers to these questions will vary with each case. It may be impossible to make a final decision until there has been an opportunity to unpick any bound-up iris tissue at the time of surgery. An algorithm for the assessment of pupil problems is presented in Scheme 3.1.

STRUCTURES AVAILABLE FOR IOL IMPLANTATION

Pseudophakia usually offers the best visual rehabilitation for reconstructed eyes. At the time of the initial examination it may be possible to assess the most appropriate fixation method for IOL implantation. The preferred order of choice, with the structures required, are listed in Table 3.4.

Even if there is sufficient capsular material for a sulcus-fixated lens, it may be enmeshed with iris and vitreous. This will need to be dissected free early on in the surgical procedure, hence a final decision on IOL fixation may only be possible per-operatively.

Calculation of lens power requires biometry. In some cases this will be impossible or inaccurate in the damaged eye, hence keratometry and axial length measurements from the healthy eye should be used.

PATHOLOGY PRECLUDING A GOOD VISUAL OUTCOME

Apart from the psychophysical assessments of vision mentioned above, the potential for vision can be assessed by the clinical appearance of the retina and optic nerve. Retinal commotio, detachment, haemorrhage and oedema can all degrade the final image. Trauma can lead to a macu-

Table 3.4. Structures required for IOL implantation.

Position for IOL	Structure required
Intra-capsular (in the bag)	Intact posterior capsule and zonules
Sulcus-fixated	Anterior or posterior fringe capsular diaphragm extending for a minimum of 180 degrees
Iris-sutured	Sufficient iris tissue areas diametrically opposite to each other to support lens
Scleral-sutured	Healthy sclera

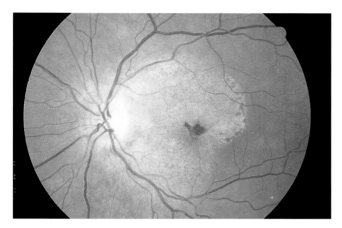

Figure 3.23. Traumatic neuropathy.

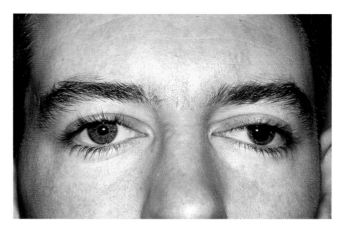

Figure 3.24. Left divergent squint.

lar hole (Fig. 3.23). Due to the chronic nature of some of these cases, in conjunction with low-grade uveitis, cystoid macular oedema is relatively common. Its presence may need to be confirmed by retinal topography or fluoroscein angiography.

Traumatic optic neuropathy may result from disruption of the vasa nervorum or from damage to the nerve itself. Compression of the nerve by a retrobulbar mass (haemorrhage or abscess) may cause optic nerve head swelling (see Chapter 2).

ANTICIPATED COMPLICATIONS

Pre-existing pathology may compromise the final outcome. A careful pre-operative examination will help you to accurately predict post-operative problems and formulate a realistic prognosis.

Strabismus

Whilst a history of a prior squint is important, a careful assessment of ocular movements should be performed to identify any subclinical eye movement abnormalities. A pre-existing divergent squint may lead to post-operative diplopia, which may be perceived by the patient as a failure, despite the surgeon's best reconstructive efforts (Fig. 3.24). Extra-ocular muscle imbalance may result from a blow-out fracture complicating the initial trauma.

Lids

Cicatricial lid or conjunctival scarring, and staphylococcal blepharitis, with any associated dryness, may lead to significant ocular surface problems (Fig. 3.25). Advanced or complex reconstructive surgery, including penetrating keratoplasty, is doomed to failure if the conjunctival and corneal epithelia are unhealthy.

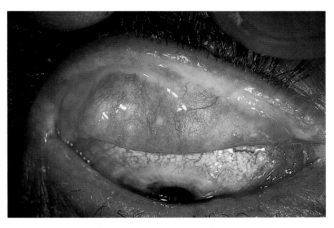

Figure 3.25. Aggressive, severe staphylococcal lid disease.

Glaucoma

Pre-operative raised intraocular pressure (IOP) frequently complicates eyes coming for reconstruction. The causes of this are listed in Table 3.5.

Post-operative raised IOP is common (see Chapter 5). If pre-operatively problems are recognized, prophylactic measures to reduce the rise after surgery can be taken (i.e. the use of topical or systemic medication).

Medical management may be required using topical or parenteral anti-hypertensive agents. The presence of glau-

Table 3.5. Causes of glaucoma in eyes coming for anterior segment reconstruction.

- Steroid responder
- Peripheral anterior synechiae causing angle closure
- Hypertensive uveitis
- Angle damage with anterior chamber IOL
- Cyclodialysis secondary to mechanical trauma
- Ghost-cell glaucoma secondary to vitreous haemorrhage

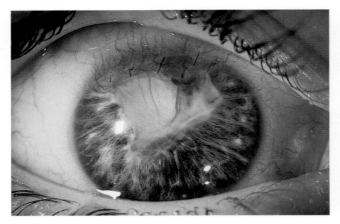

Figure 3.26. Cyclitic membrane.

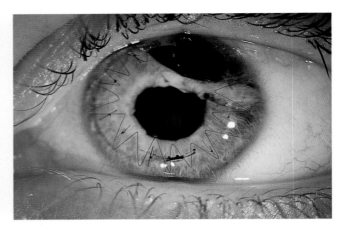

Figure 3.27. Iridodialysis.

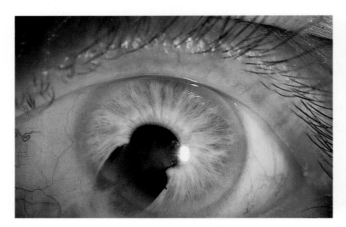

Figure 3.28. Sector iris loss.

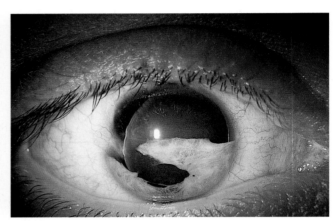

Figure 3.29. Sub total iris loss.

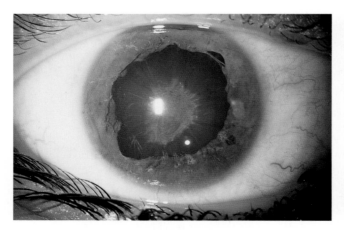

Figure 3.30. Complete sphincter rupture.

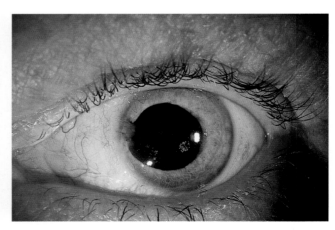

Figure 3.31. Sector sphincter rupture.

Scheme 3.1: Assessment of iris and pupillary damage.

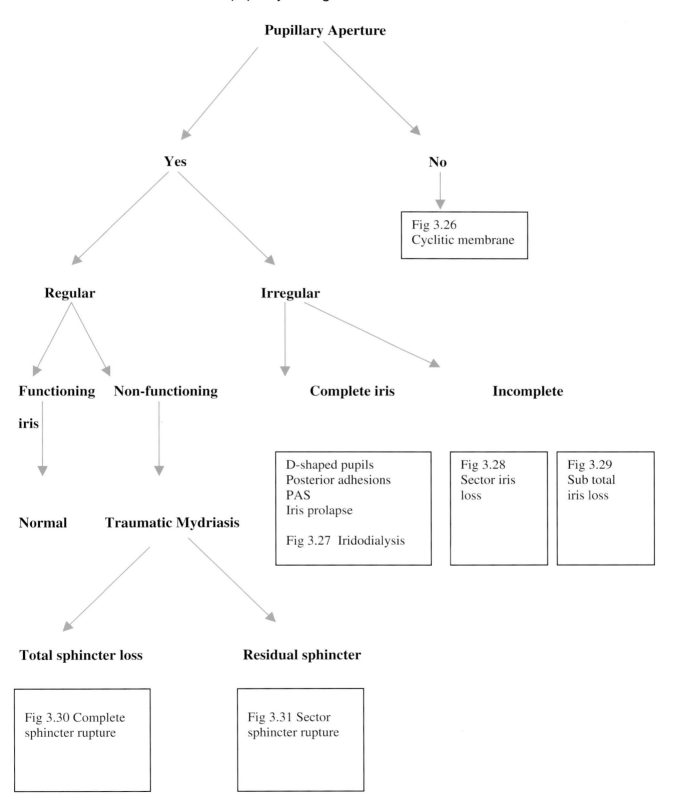

coma in an eye requiring a corneal graft is a serious concern which may require surgical intervention in the form of a standard or augmented trabeculectomy.

Patients suffering extraneous trauma involving the midsegment may have conjunctival scarring which may complicate any planned drainage procedure. In these circumstances, a tubal implant may be indicated.

Uveitis

The patient may have pre-existing uveitis as a primary condition, irrespective of the inflicted damage. Anterior chamber inflammation may be caused by the original injury, e.g. a mis-sized anterior chamber lens or herniating vitreous. Inflammation of the posterior segment may lead to cystoid macular oedema which may have permanent effects on visual potential. Uveitis may be one of the causes of raised IOP.

INVESTIGATIONS

If there is some doubt regarding the aetiology of a given traumatic event, and especially where it is impossible to visualize the posterior segment, alternative imaging modalities can be used to determine the integrity of those parts of the eye which cannot be seen.

Ultrasonography can benefit the surgeon in a number of ways. A-scanning will allow objective assessment of the axial lengths of both eyes. If IOL implantation is required, it may be impossible to accurately judge the appropriate power from axial length measurements of the damaged eye. With no history of amblyopia (which can be anisometropic in origin) it is often better to use the axial length of the fellow eye for calculation purposes. A reduced axial length, noted on A-scanning, may be indicative of a silent posterior globe rupture. B-scanning, with image capture

printing, allows dynamic and static visualization of the vitreous, retina and sclera (and any IOFBs that may be present).

Imaging, using plain X-rays, CT or MRI scans, may be required in cases of adnexal damage or bone trauma where orbital integrity may have been compromised. Radiological investigation can pin-point an orbital foreign body (Fig. 3.32).

Before drawing up a final therapeutic plan to offer to the patient, you must have a clear idea in your own mind of any surgery that may be required. Each of the tissues must be considered independently, assessing the need for extension, replacement, reconstruction, or artificial exchange. Once the sum of these steps has been 'calculated', a surgical plan, spread over one or several operations, may be presented.

The next chapter discusses the principles of the surgical techniques employed in reconstructive anterior segment surgery.

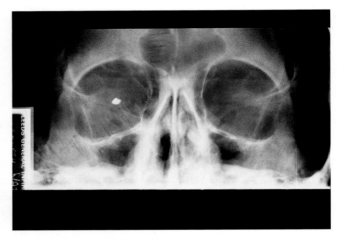

Figure 3.32. Metallic foreign body in the optic nerve.

Chapter 4

Reconstructive techniques

INTRODUCTION

The normal function and anatomy of the eye will be disrupted by any traumatic insult to the eye. These effects have to be appreciated and managed. Tissues which have been lacerated or bruised will scar as they heal, joining together structures which are normally independent of each other. The contraction of these fibrotic elements, compounded by the splinting effect of prolapsed vitreous, will hold the damaged tissues together, distorting the pupil and entrapping the normally mobile iris. A fibrovascular, pupillary membrane may contract, disinserting the ciliary body or pull on the vitreous base and cause a retinal detachment. When the cause of the disorganization was a surgical complication, a misplaced and incarcerated IOL may also be found.

These complex processes, frequently involving many tissues, will continue to cause damage unless the surgical interception fully addresses the pathological processes.

The aims of reconstructive surgery are to realign the eye's anatomical elements into their correct positions and thereby to restore vision. By refashioning a pupil, e.g. from the remnants of the iris and capsule, or by correcting a squint by surgery or injecting botulinum toxin, a patient's appearance may be greatly improved.

Reconstruction may require more than one operation and therefore it is important to remember that the last stage of one operation may be the first step for any subsequent surgical procedure. Nowhere is this more important to remember than during the execution of a primary repair when conservation and careful handling of tissue can make subsequent restorative work easier to achieve. Anticipation and planning are crucial disciplines, and this chapter will demonstrate, through worked examples of actual cases, how these principles can be applied.

PREPARATION AND ANTICIPATION

Instrumentation

The instruments required must be thought about in advance. The surgical plan for any particular patient should be discussed with the theatre staff soon enough to permit an opportunity to collect together any special tools. Reconstruction operations may not be part of the regular theatre routine, but all the tools should be easily acquired with adequate warning. The surgeon must be prepared to borrow from cataract, retinal or corneal trays, extemporizing and perhaps adapting established instruments for new uses.

The instruments recommended below reflect the authors' own preferences and experience, although every surgeon will have their own favourite hand-tools. The key instruments, which have been highlighted with an asterisk (*), have been found to make reconstructive surgery easier. They are readily available, often simple, always versatile and can be used in many situations. The instruments tend to be generic designs and similar patterns are likely to be found on any microsurgical tray.

KNIVES (Fig. 4.1)

*Fine 45° diamond blade
20-gauge MVR blade (for pars plana vitrectomy)
*Corneal trephines, various sizes, especially Hessberg–Barron disposable trephines (Fig. 4.2)
Myringotomy knife
15° angled disposable superblade
21- to 25-gauge hypodermic needles

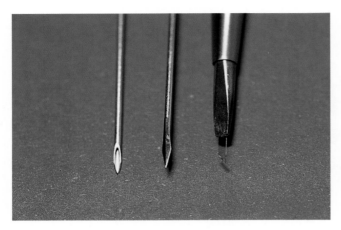

Figure 4.1. Knives from left to right: 21-gauge needle, goniotomy knife, diamond.

A diamond blade is a fundamental requirement for effective reconstructive surgery. It allows the construction of regular and precise incisions even in the most difficult circumstances, for instance in a soft eye. It can also be used to make stab corneal incisions and for cutting lammellar flaps for transclerally sutured lenses and corneal buttons, when a graft is required. Myringotomy or goniotomy knives, perhaps introduced through a stab incision,

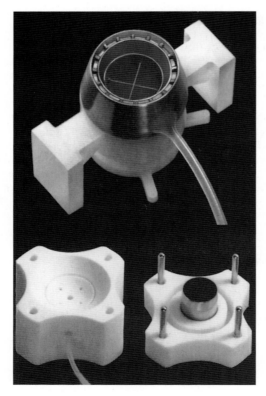

Figure 4.2. Hessburg–Barron trephine (Katena Products Inc.).

can be used to tease apart lamellae and scar tissue within an eye. The authors found them especially useful for cutting the binding adhesions which may be locking the haptics of an IOL in the anterior chamber angle.

SCISSORS (Fig. 4.3)

Extra-ocular	*Westcott's spring scissors
	*Vanna's – short- and long-bladed
Graft	Corneal graft scissors – Castroviejo's, etc.
Intraocular	*Ong's (long)
	Grieshaber's scissors with rotatable blades
	de Wekker's
	Vanna's (short and long)

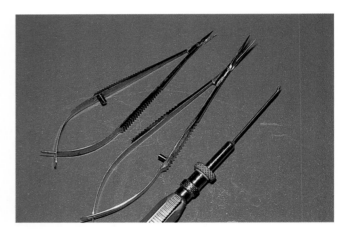

Figure 4.3. Scissors, from left to right; Vanna's, Long Ong's, Grieshaber's.

Note that these are all spring scissors. They make fine manoeuvring possible even for the most delicate intraocular dissection and can be used equally easily by right- and left-handed surgeons. Both Westcott's and Vanna's are useful in conjunctival dissection.

Long Ong's scissors are able to pass through a small corneal incision and will reach across the eye to cut tissues on the diametrically opposite side of the anterior chamber. They may be used to define and separate the leaves of the iris from scar tissue and the remnants of lens capsule. Passed gently behind the iris, snags and adhesions can be recognized and divided to allow insertion of an IOL into the ciliary sulcus (Fig. 4.4).

Angled Grieshaber's scissors with rotatable blades theoretically give access to the most difficult recesses in the anterior chamber (Fig. 4.5) but in practice they are disappointing in their performance. They are more valuable in posterior segment surgery where the surgeon is less limited by the volume of the surgical field. They are ideal for reaching down to the retinal surface and working through the small incisions of the pars plana.

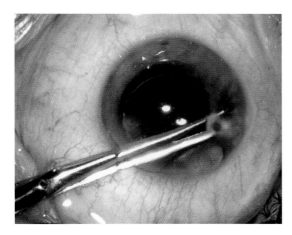

Figure 4.4. Long Ong's being used to cut anterior iris adhesion.

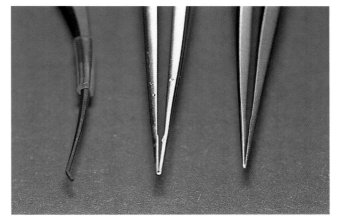

Figure 4.6. Forceps from left to right; Colibris, Pierce Hoskin's straight, tying.

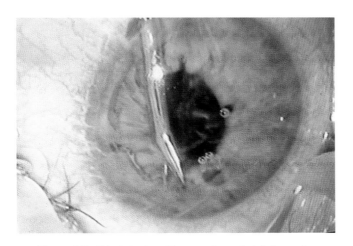

Figure 4.5. Grieshaber's cutting scar tissue in inferior angle.

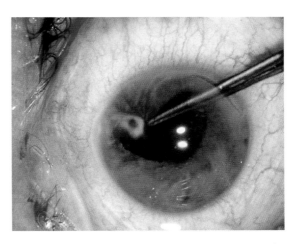

Figure 4.7. Utrata's holding iris during pupillary reconstruction.

FORCEPS (Fig. 4.6)

Extra-ocular	Jayle's, Lister's, St Martin's
Corneal and wound	*microgroove forceps with tying platforms, e.g. Pierce Hoskin's derivatives *Colibri's (Osborn & Simmons) toothed or microgroove with tying blocks
Intraocular	*Utrata's forceps (fine and long) *McPhearson's forceps (fine)

The microgroove and Colibri's forceps are ideal for corneal surgery. The slightly hooked nose of the Colibri's allows tissue to be held in a variety of different orientations. They are both available with tying blocks behind their tips.

For holding tissues within the eye, the delicate unmodified tips of McPhearson's and Utrata's forceps are invaluable (Fig. 4.7). Sometimes considerable but stable force will be needed within the anterior chamber, e.g. during manipulation or removal of an incarcerated IOL, and McPhearson's forceps are particularly recommended. Unlike the Utrata's forceps, which have slightly blocked tips, the even apposition of the McPhearson's forceps allows the slippery haptic of an intraocular lens to be firmly but gently grasped as it is manipulated. They can also double up as needle holders when suturing within the anterior chamber. They are able to grasp, guide and manipulate the minute 3.5 mm microvascular needle within the eye, holding both needle and iris as required.

NEEDLE HOLDERS

*Micro-locked/unlocked
*Noble's Ultra (Osborn & Simmons)

The very fine Noble's Ultra needle holders, produced by Osborn & Simmons, are approximately half the size of a normal micro needle holder and can be used to pass and hold a needle within the eye (Fig. 4.8). Their slim form makes it possible to rotate this needle holder within the constraints of the anterior chamber, even when limited by the short corneal wound.

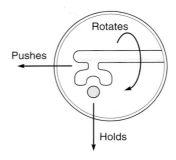

Figure 4.10. The versatility of the Kuglen hook.

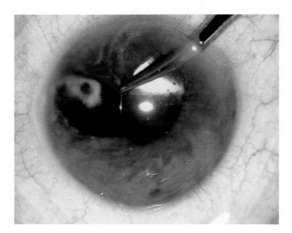

Figure 4.8. Noble's Ultra needle holder used for iris suturing.

HOOKS (Fig. 4.9)

*Kuglen
*Sinskey
Grieshaber iris retractors

The Kuglen hook is designed to push, pull and hold tissues or to manipulate the trailing haptic of an intraocular lens. The different facets on its surface make it particularly versatile (Fig. 4.10). The Sinskey, which is the simplest hook, is a particularly gentle probe that may be used to define and divide adhesions between iris, vitreous and capsule and may also be bent into a useful shape to cope with a difficult dissection in an awkward angle. Other bespoke

hooks can be easily made by bending hypodermic needles or the tips of Rycroft cannulae.

Grieshaber iris retractors are particularly valuable in phacoemulsification or pars planar vitrectomies when a small pupil has to be held open. In reconstructive surgery, the hooks can be used to hold flaccid iris or unstable capsule.

VITRECTOMY EQUIPMENT

Guillotine suction cutter: Alcon Accurus, Oertli, Ocutome, etc.
Pars planar infusion cannulae – regular and long (4 or 6 mm)
*Anterior chamber infusion/maintainer (Visitec) (Fig. 4.11)
Self-retaining anterior chamber maintainers of different length
*21-gauge Butterfly with artery clip (Fig. 4.12)

Vitrectomy is frequently necessary during a reconstructive operation. The surgeon must be familiar with this equipment and able to perform an anterior vitrectomy. The vitrector should have a guillotine cutter with a variable rate of cutting, levels of vacuum and an adjustable port. Inferior quality or malfunctioning equipment will cause

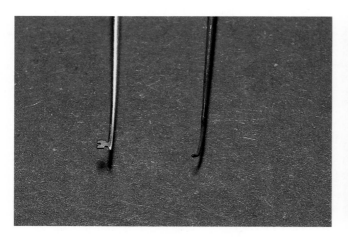

Figure 4.9. Hooks from left to right: Kuglen and Sinskey.

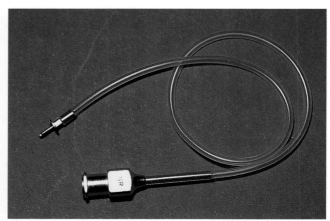

Figure 4.11. Visitec self-retaining infusion cannula.

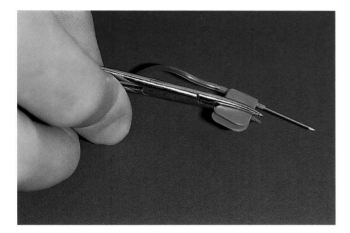

Figure 4.12. Butterfly 21-gauge is held in fine anterior clip.

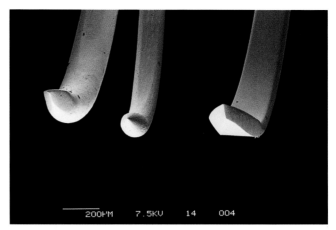

Figure 4.13. Scanning election micrographs of needle tips: taper-cut, round-bodied and CS Ultima Ethicon needles (courtesy of Mr Keith Clark, Ethicon Ltd).

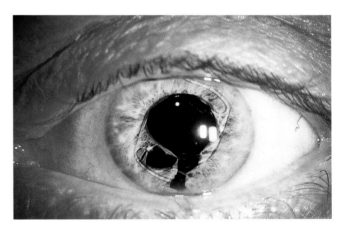

Figure 4.14. Iris laceration from spatulated needle during attempt at iris repair. This would not have happened if a round-bodied needle had been used.

vitreous traction and retinal detachment, or damage anterior segment tissues. (Other vitrectomy instrumentation, including light pipe and corneal lens, should be available but will only be needed if surgery is undertaken in the posterior segment).

The advances in the design, and ease of use, of vitreous suction cutters enable rapid and atraumatic clearance of vitreous from the anterior chamber. Rapid cutting rates should be used when removing vitreous alone (240 or more cuts per minute), but when cutting capsule or scar tissue, for instance when creating an artificial pupil or defining tissue spaces, a much slower cutting rate should be used. This gives time for the tissues to enter the cutting port prior to abscission. Take care not to inadvertently capture and amputate the iris when working close to the iris surface.

When working in the anterior chamber, a pars planar infusion line will not be required. Use instead either a self-retaining infusion cannula such as the Visitec cannulae, or if a more dynamic, bimanual approach is needed to handle or separate structures, a Butterfly cannula held in an artery clip or in the fingers is a simple but elegant alternative (see Fig. 4.12). With a hand-held infusion the stream may be directed away from the point of cutting, preventing hydration of the vitreous. It may also be used to disentangle and dissect vitreous strands incarcerated around the iris or in the port of the vitrector.

NEEDLES AND SUTURES

A variety of different needles and sutures are presented in Table 4.1. Microsurgical needles are sophisticated in design (Fig. 4.13). 'micro point' or 'spatula' needles are designed to pass easily through the lamellae of the cornea and sclera, but they will shred any delicate intraocular structures such as iris (Fig. 4.14). Conversely, round-bodied, microvascular needles will penetrate iris without tearing these delicate tissues, but are unable to penetrate sclera or cornea.

CAUTERY

*Monopolar, 'paintbrush' diathermy.
Bipolar cautery forceps (free-standing machine or via phaco/vitrectomy) machine

The Oertli intraocular diathermy may also be used if the surgeon faces a densely vascularized membrane that needs to be divided.

CANNULAE

*Disposable fine 30-gauge Rycroft (with Healon® is 27-gauge)
Viscoelastic cannulae (25- to 27-gauge)
Simcoe and McIntyre infusion/aspiration cannulae for removing viscoelastics and blood at the end of operation.

Table 4.1. Needles and sutures for anterior segment surgery. Reference numbers are all Ethicon unless stated otherwise.

1. Sclera	Needle	Length	Single/double	Reference
8-0 vicryl	Micro-point, reverse cut	8 mm		W9545
9-0 nylon	Advanced micro-point spatulated	6 mm	Double	W1769
2. Stay sutures				
4-0 Prolene	Taper-cut	17 mm		W8935
3. Corneal graft				
10-0 nylon	Side-cutting	3/8 circle	Single/Double	Alcon 208001, 198001
4. Corneal section/ wounds, incisions				
10-0 nylon	Side-cutting		As above	Alcon 208001, 198001
10-0 nylon	Advanced micro-point, spatulated 3/8 circle	6 mm, 3/8 circle	Single	W1768
11-0 nylon	As above	As above	Double	W1780
5. Iris repair				
10-0 Prolene	Round bodied	3.75 mm (75μm diameter)	Single	W2790
10-0 nylon	Round bodied	3.75 mm (75μm diameter)	Single	W2870
6. Iris/scleral sutured IOLs				
10-0 Prolene	Taper-cut	13 mm, 1/4 circle, long curved	Double	788G
10-0 Prolene	Micro-point plus	16 mm straight	Double	W1713
10-0 Prolene	Micro-point spatulated	6 mm, 3/8 circle	Double	W1710
7. Astigmatic, graft re-suture				
10-0 nylon	Bi-curve, side cut	'fish hook'	Single (double pack with 4-0 silk)	Alcon 305301
8. Limbal grafts, amniotic membrane				
10-0 vicryl	CS Ultima		Single	V960 G

The fine 30-gauge Rycroft cannulae is used to reform the anterior chamber through a corneal stab incision (note that heavy viscoelastics will not pass easily through these narrow cannulae). Larger cannulae, although useful for injecting balanced salt solution to reform the eye, let fluid escape around the cannula almost as rapidly as it is injected, making it difficult to judge whether or not a wound is watertight at the end of surgery.

VISCOELASTICS

Many viscoelastic agents are now available and each surgeon will have their own preferences. The high-molecular-weight (MW), long-chain viscoelastic agents, such as Healon® GV, may be particularly valuable in 'visco'-dissection. Although providing an excellent tamponade in the anterior chamber, it will not stay in the eye if the intraocular pressure increases or when the anterior chamber is reformed. Once the heavy MW viscoelastic begins to extrude from the eye, the whole viscoelastic bolus will

tend to follow (hence the description of 'cohesive'). In contrast, the shorter chain, lower-molecular-weight viscoelastic agent such as Healon® 5, Amvisc, Viscoat and Methylcellulose are excellent tissue space expanders, but require to be removed piecemeal at the end of the operation (these are 'dispersive'-type viscoelastic agents). These shorter molecules will give a sustained protection of the corneal endothelium, but may be difficult to remove at the end of an operation, especially after complex microsurgical dissection and repair.

FLUIDS

Balanced salt solution (BSS) (either 'plus' or 'standard'). Adrenaline (intracardiac) at 10^{-6} (one in a million) concentration is routinely added to the infusion to help maintain dilatation of the pupil. These physiological infusion fluids have established roles in phacoemulsification and vitrectomy.

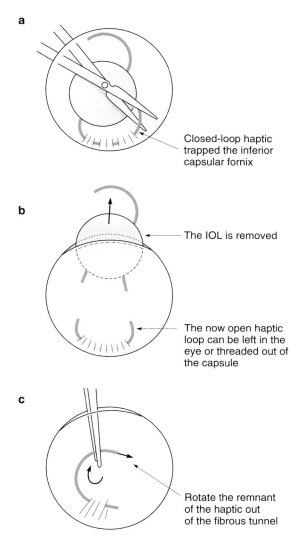

a

Closed-loop haptic trapped the inferior capsular fornix

b

The IOL is removed

The now open haptic loop can be left in the eye or threaded out of the capsule

c

Rotate the remnant of the haptic out of the fibrous tunnel

Figure 4.24. (a–c) Removal of closed-loop IOL with inferior haptic adhesions. (a) Vanna's scissors are used to cut close to the optic/haptic junctions. (b) The optic is removed leaving the inferior haptic buried in its adhesions. (c) The inferior haptic is 'dialled' out of its adhesions.

Without the restrictions of the optic and its other attachments, the cut loop will be easily released.

Silicone plate haptics should be approached slightly differently. Holes in the plate haptics are quickly penetrated by dense fibrosis and the rubbery nature of the lens makes them difficult to cut. Make the corneal incision at right angles to the long axis of the lens and then separate the IOL from the posterior surface of the capsule by injecting viscoelastic (Figs 4.25a and b). Carefully pass the tip of the long Ong's scissors through the capsulorrhexis and divide the adhesions. The IOL will pop out into the AC, and can be quickly removed from the eye.

Acrylic lenses (e.g., Acrysoft) seem to lie within the capsule and inhibit anterior to posterior capsular adhesions.

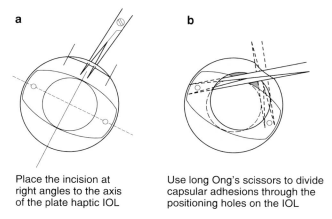

a

Place the incision at right angles to the axis of the plate haptic IOL

b

Use long Ong's scissors to divide capsular adhesions through the positioning holes on the IOL

Figure 4.25. (a and b) Removal of a silicone plate IOL. The orientation of the incision is crucial to enable division of adhesions through positioning holes.

This means that it is possible to completely reopen the capsular bag. When exchanging these lenses, spin the lens around fully opening the bag. The replacement IOL can then be placed into this ideal position.

(2) Lenses in the posterior segment

IOLs lying free in (or falling into) the vitreous present their own problems. If a lens is lying on the retina or in the posterior vitreous an anterior segment surgeon should not attempt to remove or replace this without the help of a vitreo-retinal colleague. A decision may be made to leave the lens where it rarely causes any problems to the retina. The major visual difficulty reported by patients is that they notice, first thing in the morning, a circular shadow in their vision. Once the patient is up and about, the lens will fall inferiorly and move out of notice.

If the lens is visible in the anterior vitreous, it can be carefully caught with a hook and held in place whilst an anterior vitrectomy is carried out, freeing the lens from all vitreous attachments before it is taken from the eye (Figs 4.26a–c and 4.27). Sometimes the eye will have to be gently moved from side to side to get a good view of it, but there is no place for 'blind fishing' in the posterior segment in an attempt to stir up the vitreous and 'find' the IOL. This is extremely dangerous and runs a high risk of damaging the retina or disturbing the vitreous.

(3) Removing AC IOLs

Earlier designs of AC IOLs had either closed-loop haptics (Azar B lens) or positioning holes. Angle adhesions were frequently extensive and associated with aggressive fibrosis. Removing these lenses is potentially hazardous because of the risk of iris root disinsertion and catastrophic

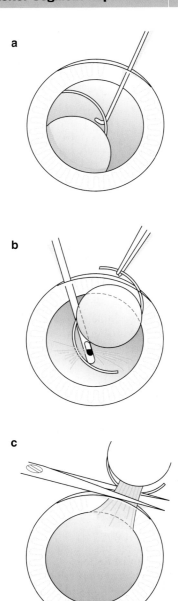

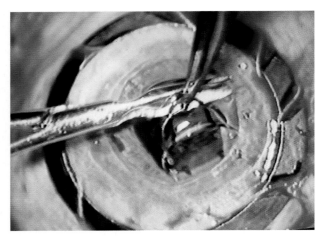

Figure 4.27. A Binkhorst iris-clip lens is removed from the anterior vitreous in an eye during a corneal graft. Note that all vitreous adhesions are divided before the lens is lifted out of the eye.

(4) Iris and pupil

When defining the tissue planes of the anterior segment, every effort should be made to conserve as much iris tissue as possible. This will help with both the function and cosmetic appearance of the eye as well as potentially providing support for an IOL. It may be possible to repair the iris, but if there is very little left, an IOL incorporating an artificial pupil (and a coloured haptic) might be used. Artificial pupil lenses, such as the Morcher system, may help stop-down the amount of light entering the eye, but, because they are incapable of reacting, do not necessarily reduce the symptoms of glare (Figs 4.30–4.33).

(5) Lens

Usually these eyes are already aphakic or pseudophakic but after either blunt or perforating trauma, the natural lens may still be in situ. If a cataract is forming it will be necessary to remove the lens, using a capsule tension ring if there has been any damage to the zonule. After a perforating injury, either or both anterior and posterior capsules may have been pierced and an anterior vitrectomy may then be needed (an ultrasound should help diagnose a through-and-through lens injury, pre-operatively). Retain any capsular fringe if at all possible; sulcus fixation is preferable to any sort of sutured fixation for the IOL.

Figure 4.26. (a–c) Removal of IOL from the anterior vitreous. Use of the Sinskey hook to capture a haptic. Pull the haptic into the anterior chamber and cut around the posterior surface of the lens with a vitrector. As the lens is delivered from the eye, cut any remaining strand of vitreous with a pair of long-bladed scissors. Complete the anterior vitrectomy.

haemorrhage. Having made the incision into the eye, gentle probing of the haptics will show whether they will be easily released. If in doubt, it is safer to cut and leave the haptic behind, removing only the optic (Figs 4.28a–d). A goniotomy knife can be used, with a fenestrated Koeppe goniolens, to cut angle adhesions (Fig. 4.29). The technique is difficult and it is simpler to leave the haptic behind.

RESTORING VISUAL FUNCTION

To see, an eye has to have a clear pathway for light (transparent cornea, clear pupil and vitreous), and an intact retina. Vision is enhanced by the presence of some sort

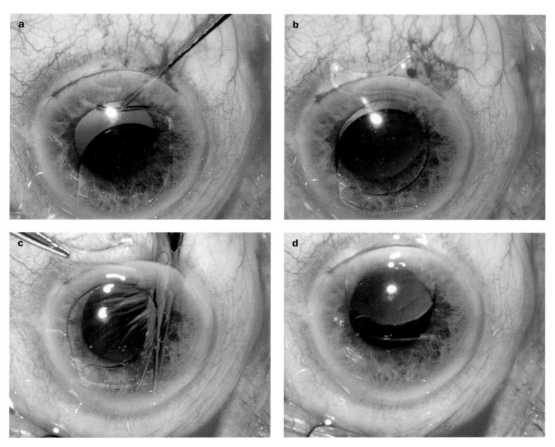

Figure 4.28. (a–d) Removal of an AC IOL with incarcerated vitreous and chronic uveitis. The upper loop of a Multiflex lens is easily dislodged from the angle and delivered through the section. The lower haptic was unyielding. Straight Vanna's scissors are used to cut it from the optic. Leaving this distal fragment behind, the remainder of the lens is removed.

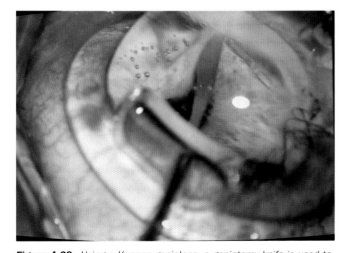

Figure 4.29. Using a Koeppe goniolens, a goniotomy knife is used to cut angle adhesions.

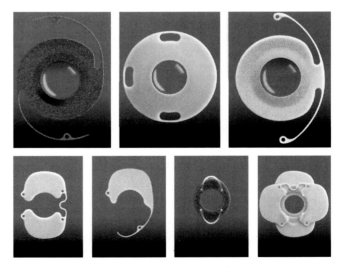

Figure 4.30. Artificial pupil system- Ophthec BV, (courtesy of Vision Matrix, Knaresborough, UK).

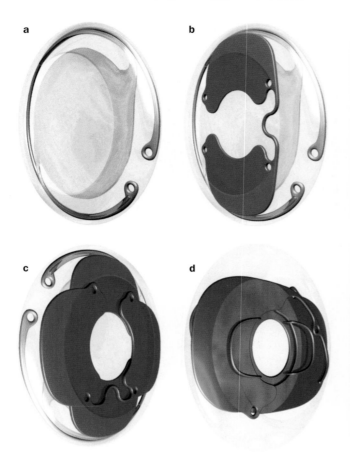

Figure 4.31. (a–d) Iris defects can be occluded by inserting a series of plates into the capsule until an artificial iris diaphragm is created. The capsule must be intact to use this system. (Courtesy of Vision Matrix, Knaresborough, UK).

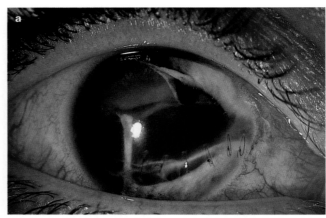

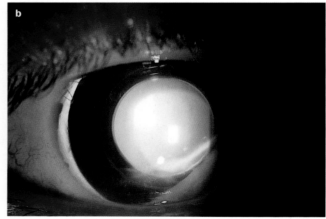

Figure 4.32. (a and b) Morcher lens, with black haptic, successfully blocks excess light in an eye with traumatic aniridia (slit lamp and red reflex photographs).

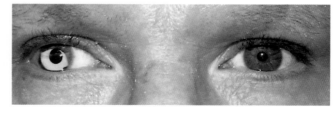

Figure 4.33. The colour of this painted haptic is too light for this patient causing cosmetic embarassment.

of pupil to stop-down the light (iris repair or artificial pupil) and improve depth and quality of focus; and a lens of optimal power (secondary lens implantation). Contact lenses and spectacles have their place in refining visual performance, and the patient must accept that they may also be needed as part of the process of visual rehabilitation.

(1) Corneal grafting

Significant endothelial cell loss, occurring during the primary trauma, is well described by many authors. As a result, transient corneal oedema often follows repair of a primary injury and, later, may be remembered as the harbinger of future corneal decompensation.

When using an open-sky approach use a scleral support band, whether Flieringa's Ring (Figs 4.34a and b) or Micra Scleral Support Band. This will reduce the tendency of the globe to distort and collapse following anterior vitrectomy

or extended mainipulations; it also helps improve accuracy when suturing the corneal button in place.

ROTATING AUTOGRAFT

The possibility of using a rotating corneal autograft should always be considered, particularly in children. The postoperative course is usually simple. The tissues heal quickly and do not need the clinical surveillance of an

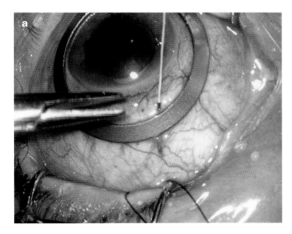 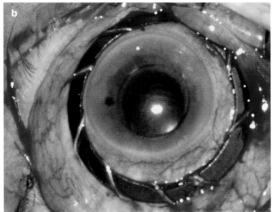

Figure 4.34. (a) Scleral support band is sutured in place with 5-0 Dacron. (b) Scleral support band – ready for cutting button.

allograft. The steroid requirements are much less. When offering this type of graft, it has to be remembered that the cornea may have already suffered significant endothelial damage, and that long-term survival may be reduced.

Interestingly, the scar will tend to clear when it is rotated away from any vascularized pedicle. If, or when, a secondary (allo)graft is later needed, the eye will be quieter, and grafting easier.

If there is a small or central opacity and the peripheral cornea is clear, a series of simple drawings will demonstrate whether a rotational graft is possible or not. The graft is cut eccentrically so that any scar is rotated away from the visual axis. If in doubt a penetrating keratoplasty can always be done.

TECHNIQUE FOR ROTATIONAL AUTOGRAFTING

The trephine is placed so that the button is cut eccentrically, and when the button is rotated, the opacity is moved to the periphery and the clear cornea into the visual axis. Some thought is needed to work out just how any particular graft will have to be placed to achieve this. Because the graft is usually eccentric, recess the limbal conjunctiva in the area of closest apposition of the button to the limbus, to help secure good bites for the sutures. See Figs 4.35a–c and the following worked example for a summary of the procedure and clinical photographs.

PENETRATING KERATOPLASTY (ALLOGRAFT OR AUTOGRAFT)

The size of the corneal button removed should be large enough to remove any central scar and perform any surgical manoeuvres without difficulty. A corneal button of 7.5 mm (minimum) is usually sufficient. If the button is less than 7 mm, astigmatism will be induced, spoiling the visual return. If the cornea is generally opaque, e.g. in a case of bullous keratopathy, the donor button should not be less

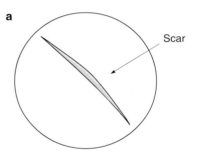

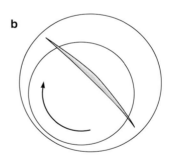

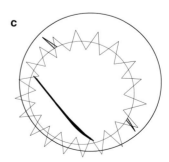

Figure 4.35. (a–c) Technique for rotational autografting. (a) Oblique scar running through the visual axis of the cornea. (b) Host button is cut eccentrically. (c) The button is rotated through 180 degrees to create a scar-free visual axis.

Worked Example 4.1

Case
A 33-year-old agricultural worker was under a tractor, chipping rust from the exhaust, when the chisel he was using fell, blade first, into his left eye.

Clinical findings
He presented 3 years after the original injury with visions of 6/6 right and CF left. The eye was quiet but had extensive fibrosis of the remaining lens capsule. There was an oblique corneal scar running through the visual axis (WE 4.1a).

Reconstruction
An eccentric corneal button was cut, allowing access to the anterior chamber. The membrane and residual capsule were carefully dissected away. This left an obvious iris defect. A Morcher artificial pupil lens was fixated to the sclera (WE 4.1b) and the corneal button was replaced, having been rotated by 180 degrees. This allowed clear cornea to be centred on the visual axis (WE 4.1c).

Outcome
Post-operative vision was 6/6-2 unaided at 2 years.

Learning points
(i) A linear corneal scar running through the visual axis can be managed with a rotational autograft.
(ii) An artificial-pupil IOL can reduce the glare and photophobia associated with large iris defects.

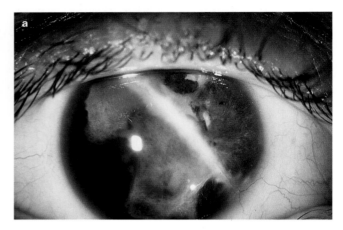

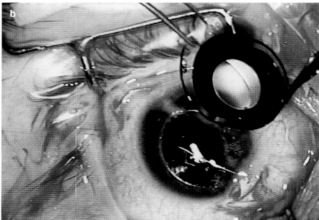

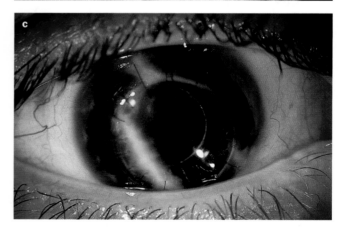

WE 4.1. (a) Linear corneal scar and dense membrane in the injured eye. (b) The corneal button and membrane have been removed and the Morcher lens is implanted. (c) Completion of the rotational autograft with clear cornea in the visual axis.

than 8 mm, with a range of 7.5 mm to 8.5 mm. In some eyes the corneal diameter may seem to be smaller than expected and in this situation the smaller graft will have to be used. Choose a trephine of either the same size as the removed button or 0.25 mm larger. Always measure the size of the recipient defect and then choose the trephine large enough to cover the defect. Small grafts may be sufficient to cover punctures or perforations, but are not nearly as structurally stable, inducing variable and high degrees of astigmatism.

TECHNIQUE

(1) The surgery is best carried out under a general anaesthetic, although a peribulbar block can also be used.

(2) A fresh or eye-banked, tissue-cultured corneo-scleral disc is used.

(3) Place stay sutures through the tendons of the vertical recti muscles; use 6-0 Prolene.

(4) Suture a scleral support band in position. Use 5-0 dacron/ethibond suture. Ensure that the band is concentric with the corneal edge.

(5) Make a paracentesis using a diamond knife and fill the eye with viscoelastic (Fig. 4.36a).

(6) Measure the diameter of the cornea and decide on the size of trephine to be used.

(7) Prepare the recipient first, cutting the button with a disposable or a Hessburg–Baron trephine, 7.5–8.5 mm in size (Fig. 4.36b). Aim to keep the corneal trephine as central as possible to keep the margins away from the edge of the cornea unless doing a rotational graft. Complete the cutting with scissors (Fig. 4.36c) or diamond blade or both. Leave the disc resting on the eye until ready to replace it with the donor button.

(8) Carry out all intraocular steps needed, including lens surgery and anterior vitrectomy.

(9) Measure the size of the hole into which the new button will be placed and choose a trephine of this size; normally this is the same size trephine as previously used.

(10) Cut the donor using the donor trephine of the Hessburg–Baron system. The corneo-scleral disc is laid endothelial side up on the vacuum cup, and covered with viscoelastic. The button is then punched whilst held in place by the vacuum (Fig. 4.36d).

(11) The recipient cornea is carefully removed and placed in a watch-glass, and covered with viscoelastic and BSS. Do not discard this until the graft is completed.

(12) The corneal button is carefully transferred to the recipient eye and sutured in place with 10-0 nylon. Four interrupted 'cardinal' sutures are inserted and then a further four. Always ensure that the sutures are placed radially and that there is sufficient viscoelastic in the eye to prevent further endothelial damage (Fig. 4.36e).

(13) Check that the eye is water-tight and then either place eight more interrupted stitches or run a continuous stitch of 10-0 nylon around the graft–host interface. Check that the sutures are all equally tight, inflate the eye with BSS, remove all viscoelastic, and bury all the knots. No knot should be proud on the corneal surface (Fig. 4.36f shows all sutures in place).

(14) A subconjuctival injection of antibiotic (cefuroxime, 125 mg) and an orbital floor or subconjunctival injection of steroid (betamethasone, 4 mg) is given. Cover the eye with a plastic shield and pad. If the surgery has been complex a prophylactic injection of intravenous (IV) acetozolamide (250 mg) is given.

(2) Pupil reconstruction

Loss of iris tissue and pupil function has serious optical effects on the eye. Depth of focus is markedly reduced, there is no adaptation to changing light intensities and glare constantly reminds the patient of their injury. Furthermore, loss of the iris and pupil produces a cosmetic blemish immediately obvious to a casual observer. Efforts to restore or re-create an iris diaphragm and some sort of pupil are therefore important objectives. Improvement in both function and appearance will result – see also the section on treatment of cosmetic issues later in this chapter.

(A) ASSESSING THE EXISTING IRIS

After injury, the iris may appear to be intact and functioning normally; it may be absent; it may be so dilated that it is virtually invisible or there may be segmental loss. The iris may be bundled-up by fibrovascular scar tissue, vitreous or both. Only by meticulous dissection can one tell how much iris tissue remains. If there is pressure to restore an iris and sufficient capsule remains, but segments of iris are missing, the artificial iris system (Ophtec) or coloured Morcher with coloured iris haptic should be considered.

(B) EXPANDING AVAILABLE IRIS

Having removed any, or all, incarcerated vitreous, hold the iris remnant with Utrata's forceps in one hand and using a hook held in the other, move around the pupil margin, gently freeing any adhesions. Pull the iris gently towards the centre of the pupil and stroke the surface of the iris, breaking down fine fibrillary elements that prevent its normal movement.

If a pupil has been 'permanently' dilated, e.g. following a blunt injury, these fine surface adhesions will cause the iris to be rolled up and held peripherally. It may be almost invisible, but it is normally possible to free extensive areas by careful dissection with probe and forceps used together. Gentle exploration of the iris surface with a

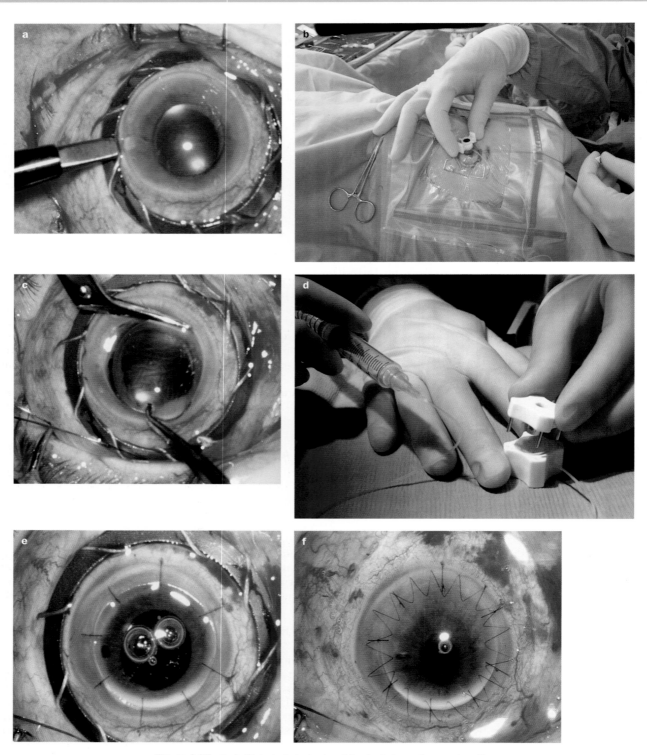

Figure 4.36. (a–f) Clinical photographs of the technique of corneal grafting.

Sinskey hook will readily demonstrate these adhesions; when a zone of adhesion is found, it may be broken down by circumferential movements of the hook, gently teasing this membrane off the surface. Use the Utrata's forceps to give counter-traction by pulling the iris margin centrally (Figs 4.37a–c).

Further freeing of iris can be achieved by cutting some of the radial iris fibres with long Ong's or Grieshaber's scissors. Again the iris margin is held with forceps and the stroma is shaved with the scissors. A ring of arrowhead-shaped stromal holes in the iris with an undisturbed pigment layer beneath will be seen but the iris will ease until there is sufficient iris for suturing, to create a pupil (Figs 4.38a and b).

(C) SUTURING THE IRIS

Closing the iris after the necessary surgical manipulations can re-create a useful pupil. More than one or two sutures

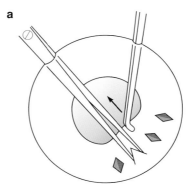

a

Further expansion of available iris can be gained by performing superficial iridotomies – cutting only the superficial stroma, leaving the pigmented layer intact

The movements are very gentle and are almost like shaving the iris

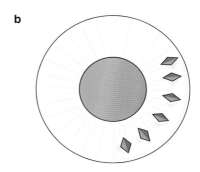

b

Figure 4.38. (a and b) Lamellar cutting of superficial iris.

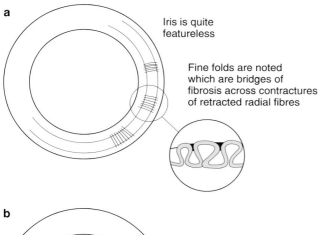

a

Iris is quite featureless

Fine folds are noted which are bridges of fibrosis across contractures of retracted radial fibres

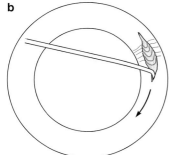

b

With a series of gentle circumferential scratching movements open up these clefts
Continue to 'recover' iris by extending the clefts with radial movements, but if too much force is used an iris dialysis may cause a sudden haemorrhage

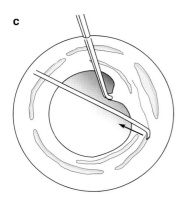

c

This technique can be used in open sky or semi-closed approaches

Figure 4.37. (a–c) The technique of freeing anterior iris adhesions using Utrata's forceps and a Sinskey hook.

may be needed to take the strain and prevent leaving a peripheral iris defect with symptoms of polycoria. The iris may be repaired as part of the IOL fixation technique in eyes without sufficient capsular support. In this way, both an iris defect can be closed and the IOL fixated by the same sutures. If scleral fixation is chosen, a separate iris repair will be required.

A series of drawings and clinical photographs will illustrate some of the options and techniques of iris suturing (Figs 4.39–4.44).

When suturing inside the anterior chamber, there is very little room to manoeuvre and the process has to be

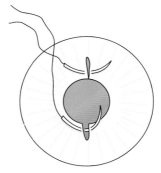

Suturing may help control very flaccid iris to produce a smaller or better shape of pupil

Figure 4.39. Suturing may help control very flaccid iris to produce a smaller or better-shaped pupil.

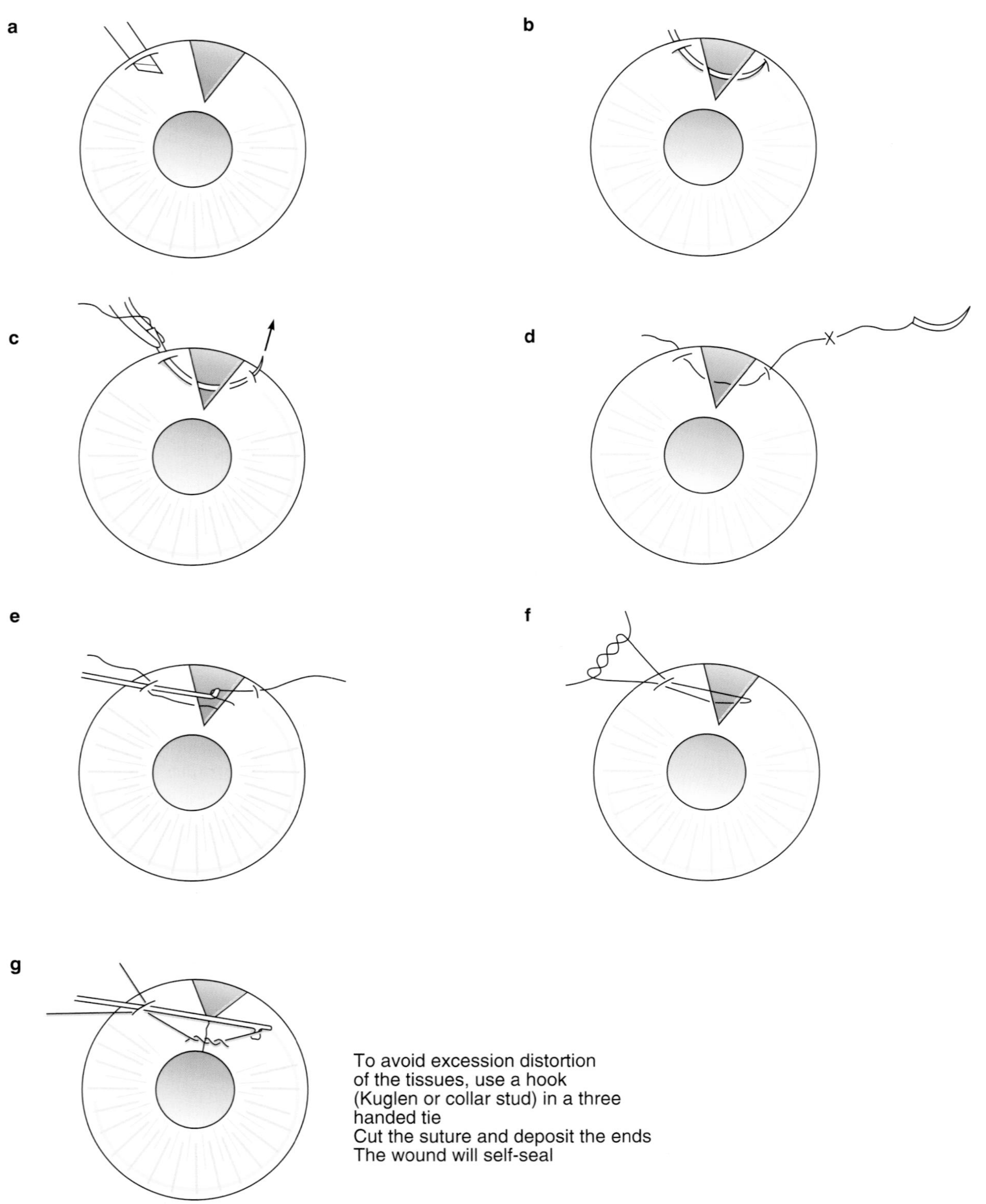

a

b

c

d

e

f

g

To avoid excession distortion
of the tissues, use a hook
(Kuglen or collar stud) in a three
handed tie
Cut the suture and deposit the ends
The wound will self-seal

Figure 4.40. (a–g) McCannel sutures – this closed-eye technique is useful for repairing peripheral iris defects. (a) A paracentesis is made close to the defect with a diamond knife. (b) Needle with 10-0 Prolene is passed through the paracentesis, and then through the iris as shown. The tip of the needle is pushed into the inner surface of the cornea to hold it in place in the AC. (c) After changing the hold on the needle, the tip is forced through the cornea. (d) The needle is cut off. (e) A hook is passed into the eye and the distal suture is retrieved and brought back out through the paracentesis. (f) The suture is tied externally and each throw of the knot is passed into the eye. (g) To avoid excessive distortion of the iris, a Kuglen hook can be used to bed down each throw of the knot (see also Figs 4.41g and h).

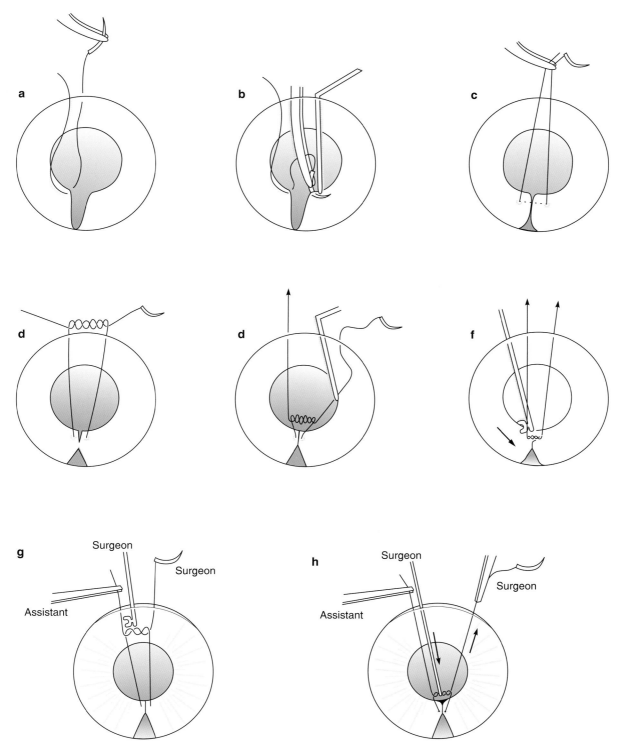

Figure 4.41. (a–f) Drawings to show the technique for internal, direct suturing of iris defects. (g,h). The three-hand tie – if it is difficult to tighten the knot inside the eye, e.g. when closing an inferior defect, a Kuglen hook can be used in a three-handed manoeuvre to achieve this. (g) One of the two arms of the 10-0 Prolene is taken by the assistant in micro-suture tying forceps and kept under gentle tension – just enough to avoid the suture becoming slack. (h) Place a Kuglen hook on the knot and slide it downwards, across the eye, to where the knot will lie. As this is done, the tension on the knot is maintained with the other hand, pulling on the slack and encouraging the hook to run smoothly to its destination.

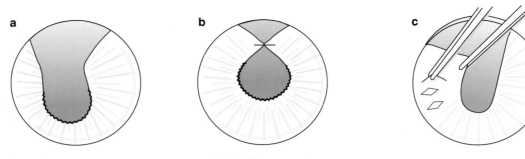

It may be possible to pass a single suture. This still leavers a large
superior coloboma – the possibility of polyopia

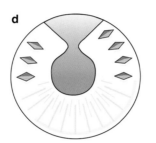

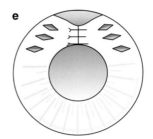

Alternatively, especially if
the defect is large, consider
implanting a Morcher style lens
with a painted haptic,
black or coloured

Figure 4.42. (a–e) Technique for closing a broad iridectomy. (a,b) It may be possible to pass a single suture to bridge the iris defect. However, this still leaves a large superior coloboma and a possibility of polyopia. (c,d) Take hold of one of the iris pillars with Utrata's forceps and create a series of superficial cuts to enhance the available iris. Do this on both sides. (e) Two or more 10-0 Prolene sutures can now be passed, giving a better repair and a smaller peripheral defect.

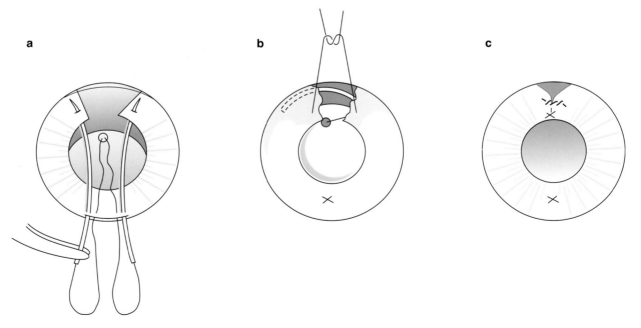

Figure 4.43. (a–c) A method of incorporating iris repair and secondary iris-sutured lens implantation. (a) Two reversed long ski-tipped needles (which are attached to the IOL through the dialling hole) are passed through the paracentesis. The base of the needles are then grasped with the needle holder and the tips passed through the proximal iris. (b) The sutures are then removed from the eye and the knots completed. (c) One or more further sutures may be placed.

broken down into its component steps. Use either McPhearson's forceps or an Ultra needle holder (Osborn and Simmons) for the tiny microvascular needle. Hold the iris with Utrata's forceps; pass the entire needle through the iris and either remove it from the eye or stick the tip into the adjacent cornea. Take hold of the distal limb of the iris, grasp the needle and once more pass it through the iris and then take it out of the eye. The knot is tied externally and the throws tightened in stages over the iris surface (Figs 4.41a–f). A three-handed tie is useful here (Figs 4.41g and h).

(D) CREATING PUPILS

Previous broad iridectomies (Fig. 4.42) and traumatic iris loss (Figs 4.43 and 4.44) can be closed to reform a pupil, either with or without secondary implantation.

The simplest surgical pupil is an optical iridectomy. This relatively old-fashioned technique was used many times to avoid cataract surgery in patients with congenital cataracts. It is a method well worth remembering, especially if microsurgical facilities are unavailable (Figs 4.45a and b). Scar tissue or capsule remnants can be used to cover a traumatic or congenital coloboma (Figs 4.46a and b). The suction-cutter can be used to give a smooth, rounded edge to this artificial pupil margin (Figs 4.47a and b). If there is a sheet of iris or scar tissue or both across the whole of the anterior chamber a central pupil can be cut with scissors or ocutome.

(E) TRAUMATIC MYDRIASIS

When the iris sphincter is damaged by a blunt injury, the iris will lie flaccid and unresponsive, but gradually contractures will form because of the unopposed action of the

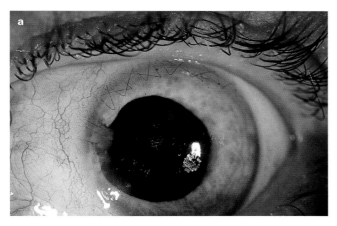
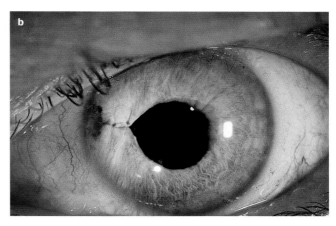

Figure 4.44. (a) Traumatic avulsion of nasal iris and lens caused by an elasticated dog lead. (b) Post-operative photograph of the same patient after treatment with a secondary lens implant and repair of the iris. Note the small peripheral defect.

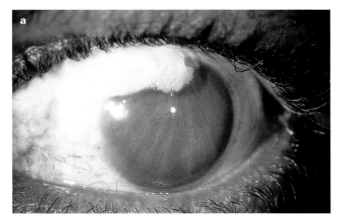
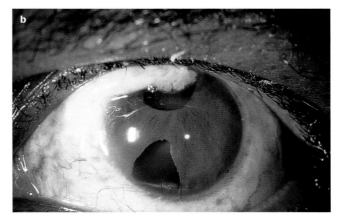

Figure 4.45. (a) A patient from the Gambia, with perception of light only, has a 'fried-egg' bleb from an irido-encleisis glaucoma operation and no apparent pupil. (b) An optical iridectomy was performed which not only created an artificial pupil but revealed the natural pupil which had been tucked behind the bleb; the vision returned to 6/18.

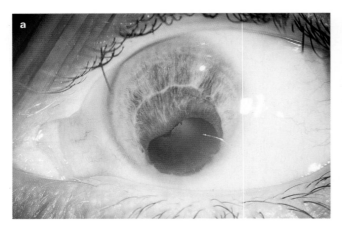
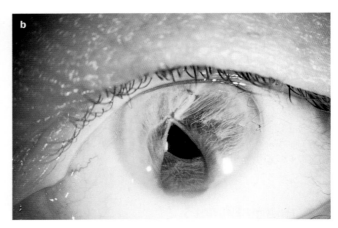

Figure 4.46. (a) A patient with microphthalmos and a congenital coloboma of iris and lens underwent extracapsular cataract surgery. A superior radial iridotomy was opened to permit the removal of a normal sized lens. (b) The radial iridotomy was partially closed with sutures, and the lower segment of the capsule with its curved capsulorrhexis provided the lower border of this central and new pupil.

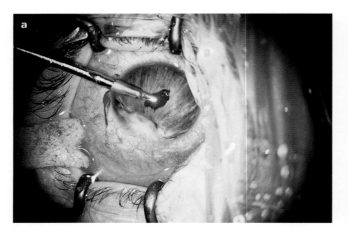
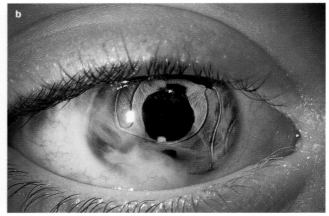

Figure 4.47. (a) This eye had suffered a serious blunt injury with partial loss of iris, lens and vitreous. A central iridotomy was made with an ocutome to create a new pupil. (b) Post-operative photograph six months later showing a white eye with a central pupil and a stable anterior chamber secondary lens.

radial muscle fibres. These will hold the pupil permanently dilated. Any attempt to produce a smaller pupil will require the division of the adhesions between the rolls of iris, and the use of sutures to maintain the reduced pupil size (Figs 4.48a and b). A closed technique may also be used by combining a series of McCannel sutures described in Figs 4.49a to f.

(F) IRIS DIALYSIS

After a blunt injury an iris dialysis may result. Late repair of such defects is difficult and often unsatisfactory because of the fibrotic changes in the iris. There is no doubt that the best time to do this is soon after the injury.

TECHNIQUE (Figs 4.50a–e)

This cleft may be repaired as follows:

(1) A flap conjunctiva and superficial sclera is lifted in the area of the dialysis.

(2) The scleral flap is gently undercut forwards to the limbus using a crescent blade (Fig. 4.50a).

(3) A counter-incision is made in the cornea on the opposite side of the eye from the dialysis (Fig. 4.50b).

(4) Fill the eye with viscoelastic and using a double-ended suture (long, straight needles, 10-0 Prolene) pass them one at a time across the eye and through the disinserted iris root. Push the needles through the angle and out under the scleral flap previously created (Figs 4.50c and d).

Table 4.6 the options for implantation in the absence of any capsular support.

Techniques

The different techniques of secondary implantation will be described, indicating the particular situations where they are most suitable.

The conjunctival sac is irrigated with 5 per cent aqueous Betadine, and the face and lids cleaned with the same. The head is draped and the lid margins covered by self-adhesive drapes. Superior and inferior rectus bridle sutures (4-0 Prolene) are inserted routinely. It is much easier to do this at the start of the operation rather than halfway through the procedure, when it is found that the eye has to be rotated into a different position.

ANTERIOR CHAMBER IOL IMPLANTATION

This technique can be used when there is insufficient capsule for sulcus fixation.

Anterior chamber implantation is the least technically demanding but needs to be done well to avoid the many problems for which the technique is infamous. It is most important to use a lens of the correct size and style. The difficulty in measuring the horizontal diameter of the cornea when the eye has had an anterior vitrectomy must be recognized. Because it is easy to underestimate the size needed, make the measurements 'prior' to opening the eye or carrying out the vitrectomy. Check the white-to-white horizontal corneal diameter and add 1 mm to get the size of the anterior chamber lens.

The choice of lens design is crucial; use a four-point fixation lens with flexible haptics, e.g. Choyce–Kelmann–Choyce style Multiflex or Clemente's three-point fixation lens. The lens should have no holes in the fixation elements of the haptics, i.e. the tips of the haptics that will sit in the angle. Avoid any lens with long trailing loops, close loops, three-piece AC IOLs or lenses with holes in their haptics. It is this group of earlier designs that is most frequently associated with complications and so they require removal.

AC IOLs should probably be reserved for older patients, where the duration of endothelial attrition will be less. Implantation is best performed as a secondary procedure because measuring the open eye for an AC IOL tends to be inaccurate. Lenses that are too big will press into the vital structures in the angle, causing chronic uveitis with accompanying pain and tenderness ('active pathology'). Vision may be compromised in the long term by cystoid macular oedema.

The possible complications of angle damage and endothelial loss makes the choice of an AC IOL a higher risk option unless the cardinal points of their use are respected.

THE TECHNIQUE OF ANTERIOR CHAMBER IMPLANTATION

Preferred lens: Alcon Multiflex MTA 3 (12.5 mm), 4 (13 mm) or 5 (13.5 mm).

(1) Measure the horizontal diameter of the cornea (white-to-white distance) and add 1 mm (Fig. 4.53a). This gives the physical size of the implant that will best fit the eye (range 11.5–13.5 mm). For example, if the white-to-white measurement is 12.5 mm, add 1 mm and the lens length needed is 13.5mm. In the Alcon style, this means that an MT5 is needed.

(2) Fill the anterior chamber with air (Fig. 4.53b).

(3) Check for vitreous strands up to the wound by sweeping with a fine cannula. Any movement or distortion of the pupil whilst doing this indicates that vitreous remains. Perform a further anterior vitrectomy if vitreous remains in the anterior chamber.

(4) Inflate the anterior chamber with viscoelastic.

(5) Pass a Sheet's lens glide into the opposite angle.

Table 4.6. Options for implantation in the absence of capsule.

Type of lens	Advantages	Possible disadvantages
1. Anterior chamber (Multiflex style)	Simplicity of technique, long-term results good	Sizing crucial, needs 2/3 iris remaining, iris incarceration, possible endothelial loss, long-term iridodenesis, cystoid macular oedema, pigment shedding, difficult to exchange
2. Iris-sutured	Anterior segment only, closed eye/open sky, iris repair can be incorporated, technically easier, uses existing IOL styles	
3. Scleral-sutured	Closed-eye/open-sky, only lens when neither iris/capsule is present, Morcher lens suitable	Technically difficult, scleral/ciliary sulcus surgery infection, ciliary body haemorrhage, cystoid macular oedema, suture fracture/dislocation, complex surgery, lens torsion/decentration, difficult to exchange

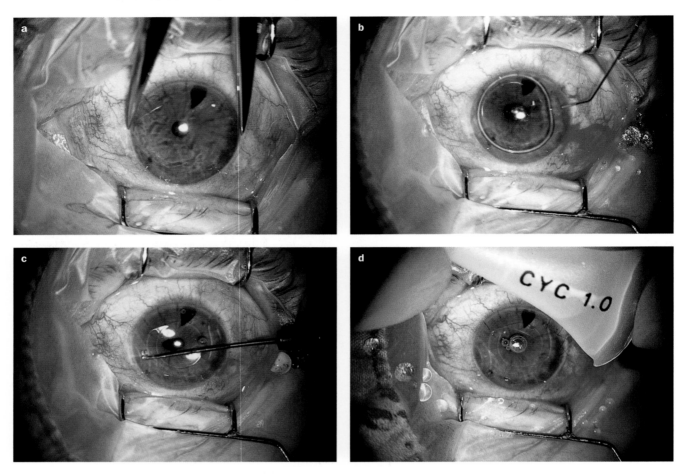

Figure 4.53. (a–d) Anterior chamber IOL implantation.

(6) Placing viscoelastic on the anterior surface of the lens glide to help the lens through the surgical wound.

(7) Insert the IOL, but aiming the legs of the lens slightly anteriorly so that iris root is kept clear of the haptic.

(8) Withdraw the lens glide.

(9) Compress the proximal loop with a Kuglen's hook, inserting the elbow and then the tip of the haptic over the lip of the corneal wound.

(10) Observe whether the pupil is round or oval; the pupil should be round and move independently when the sclera is probed. If the pupil is peaked towards one of the haptic points, the iris will have to be freed from around it. Free the iris with a Kuglen hook, by compressing the leg of the lens and lifting it slightly forwards (Fig. 4.53c). This should let the incarcerated iris slip out, and the pupil will quickly return to its round shape. (If the lens is too long, the pupil will remain oval even after the tips of the lens have been disengaged from the iris in the angle. It must be exchanged for a lens one size smaller. If it is too small, the lens will be unstable and will slip from the position it has been placed in.)

(11) Inject miochol to constrict the pupil and to check that the lens and iris are free from each other.

(12) Perform a peripheral iridectomy to avoid pupil block glaucoma.

(13) Remove any viscoelastic.

(14) Record the post-operative axis of the lens such that, at a later date in the clinic, any lens movement can be appreciated and documented.

(15) Close the corneal wound with a continuous 10-0 nylon suture.

(16) Instil Cyclopentolate 1 per cent drops to dilate the pupil (Fig. 4.53d). See also Figures 4.54 and 4.55.

SULCUS FIXATION – POSTERIOR CHAMBER LENS IMPLANTATION IN THE PRESENCE OF A CAPSULAR RIM

Where there is more than 200 degrees of capsular fringe, it is usually safe to implant an IOL into the irido-capsular sulcus. A one-piece polymelthylmethacrylate (PMMA) lens with an overall length of 13.5 mm is the preferred

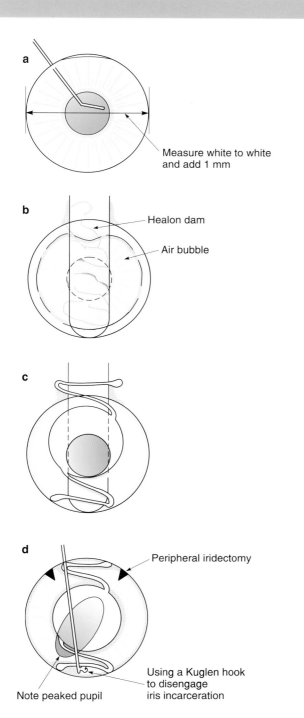

a

Measure white to white and add 1 mm

b

Healon dam

Air bubble

c

d

Peripheral iridectomy

Using a Kuglen hook to disengage iris incarceration

Note peaked pupil

Figure 4.54. (a–d) AC IOL implantantion – drawings to illustrate the cardinal steps of anterior chamber lens implantation.

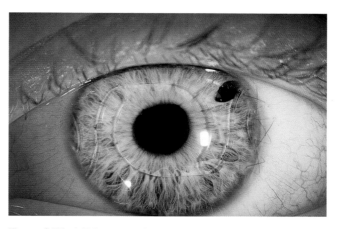

Figure 4.55. A Kelman multiflex lens satisfactorily positioned across the horizontal axis with a round, central pupil. The vision in this eye remains at 6/5, 10 years later.

ent to the iris. In more complicated cases, there may be sectors of complete capsule loss, or adhesions between the remaining capsule and iris, often splinted by the hyalinized remnants of vitreous. Sharp dissection using long Ong's scissors, Sinskey hook or a micro-vitreo-retina (MVR) blade will be needed to create sufficient sulcus for implantation.

Having identified the remaining capsule, the surgeon will also have established the optimum orientation for lens implantation. Both haptic poles must rest in the sulcus for the lens to be stable and a Sheet's glide will ensure safe delivery of the lens into the ciliary sulcus.

TECHNIQUE FOR IMPLANTING INTO THE CILIARY SULCUS

Any lens implanted into the sulcus must be at least 13 mm (better if 13.5 mm) in overall length, e.g. Bausch and Lomb 68UV, IOLAB EB33B, Alcon CVC 1U.

(1) Make a grooved corneal incision to 75 per cent of the corneal depth. The length will depend on the diameter of the optic of the lens to be used. For the recommended lens a 7.5 mm incision will suffice (see earlier).

(2) Enter the anterior chamber with a diamond-knife stab at either end of the wound.

(3) Explore the capsular remnant and its attachment to the iris. Open any adhesions with viscoelastic or hook. Delicately cut any remaining adhesions with Ong's scissors (see earlier).

(4) Identify and remove any vitreous present with a suction-cutter.

(5) Inject further viscoelastic to open the sulcus (Fig. 4.56a).

(6) Introduce a Sheet's lens glide, resting the leading edge in the opposite sulcus.

style, especially if the haptics are long. They will offer a broad, soft, circumferential attachment. During preparation of the eye for implantation the remaining capsule must be conserved, especially if an anterior vitrectomy is performed. If there is a large residual rim, lamellar dissection may be unnecessary because the capsule is often not adher-

(7) Inject viscoelastic along the upper surface of the lens glide to assist implantation.

(8) Introduce the IOL using McPhearson's forceps so that the leading haptic rests in the opposite sulcus (Fig. 4.56b).

(9) Use the Kuglen hook to flex the trailing haptic and push it into the proximal sulcus (Fig. 4.56c).

(10) Remove the viscoelastic.

(11) Inject acetylcholine to ensure that there is no pupil trapping by vitreous.

(12) Close the wound with a continuous 10-0 nylon suture (Fig. 4.56d).

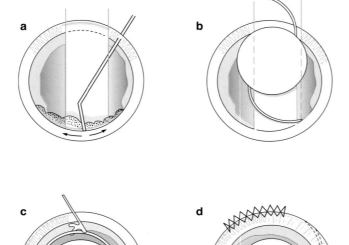

Figure 4.56. (a–d) Sulcus-fixated IOL.

IRIS FIXATION OF IOL

Posterior chamber implantation in the absence of sufficient capsule requires that the lens is either sutured to the iris or the sclera. In a situation where a surgeon wants to implant a back-up lens, and if an anterior chamber lens is not available, or there is insufficient capsule support, suturing the lens to the iris is possible even with such a soft eye.

The technique is also a useful alternative for secondary implantation, particularly if it is the intention to repair a defect in the iris.

This straightforward technique allows the secure implantation of an IOL into the posterior chamber. The lens is attached to the iris by 10-0 Prolene sutures passed

through and gently tied to the iris. The lens must have two patent dialling holes to allow the suture to be tied to it. (Note that some styles of lens have dialling notches which are not patent.) The IOL is brought up against the back surface of the iris and the sutures tied. Iridodenesis and phacodenesis are not usually seen as the haptics of the IOL find their way into the ciliary sulcus. In addition to its value in secondary implantation, this technique may be adapted to other difficult situations:

- to supplement intraocular lens implantation with iris repair
- to help closure of congenital or surgical colobomata
- to supplement sulcus fixation, if there is uncertainty about the security of the lens in the sulcus
- as a means of securing an IOL when the capsule is lost during complicated primary cataract surgery and the appropriate back-up lens is not available
- if the largest available lens is too short for the dimensions of the capsular bag or anterior chamber, e.g. in a large, myopic eye.

In these circumstances the lens can be attached to the iris without the need for the dissection of partial thickness scleral flaps, always difficult in a soft eye.

IRIS FIXATION: TECHNIQUE

Preferred lens: Bausch and Lomb 68UV, or Alcon CVC1U, or any lens with dialling holes in the optic or haptic approximately 7 mm away from each other.

Special suture: Ethicon long 'ski-tip', double-armed, on 10-0 Prolene.

The 12 to 6 o'clock meridian is the easiest axis for this type of lens implant. A suitable intraocular lens is chosen, usually with at least a 6.0 mm optic with dialling holes outside this diameter, e.g. Bausch and Lomb 68UV or CVC1U lens (Alcon). The dialling holes must be patent for the fixation of the suture to the lens.

(1) Make a grooved, 7.5 mm posterior corneal incision centred at 12 o'clock.

(2) Make a counter-stab incision with the diamond knife at 6 o'clock (Fig. 4.57a).

(3) Perform an anterior vitrectomy to clear the pupil and anterior chamber. Divide and remove other vitreous binding elements (Fig. 4.57b).

(4) With the cannula on the syringe containing the viscoelastic or Sinskey hook, investigate and clear the tissue behind the iris in an attempt to identify any capsular remnants.

(5) Place a moistened self-adhesive foam pad on the drape over the patient's forehead. This makes a safe 'work-bench' whilst carrying out the tricky steps of tying the sutures to the lens and during the implantation process.

(6) The IOL is removed from its packaging and placed on the moistened pad. Each of the long ski-tipped needles (mounted on 10-0 Prolene) is passed through the dialling hole and the pair of needles passed back through the loop in the suture; a simple slip knot results (Figs 4.57c and d). This is repeated for the opposite dialling hole.

(7) Each of the two leading needles is passed across the eye, behind the iris, and then through the peripheral iris, about two-thirds of the way between the pupil margin and the edge of the visible iris. Leave a gap of approximately 2 mm between the iris punctures, sufficient for tying the sutures across (Fig. 4.57e).

(8) Each needle is guided through the pre-placed stab incision at 6 o'clock by docking its tip in the mouth of a Rycroft cannula, pushed through the stab incision (this prevents the tip of the long needle from catching the Descemet's membrane).

(9) The lens is placed in the eye, simultaneously drawing on the Prolene threads which pull the lens optic into its final resting place (and possibly pulls the haptics into the ciliary sulcus) (Fig. 4.57f). Cut off the distal needles and after placing one throw in the Prolene, tighten this gently onto the iris surface.

(10) A hook is swept across the distal anterior chamber to check that Descemet's membrane has not been snagged by the suture. The suture is carefully laid to the side and out of the way of the next suturing steps.

(11) The upper haptic is now passed into the eye and, using a Kuglen hook, pushed behind the iris superiorly (pushing the haptic into the eye by pronating the hand, as in conventional implantation, runs the risk of damaging the iris and compromising the security of the implant). The upper half of the lens now hangs backwards in the eye.

(12) The upper sutures are now passed through the upper iris. Take the 'tip' of the needle in the needle holder and pass the 'reverse end' of the needle across the anterior chamber, but this time in front of the iris (Fig. 4.57g). Again dock this into the Rycroft cannula and draw it partially through the stab incision.

(13) The rear of the needle is then grasped with a needle holder and passed back (tip first) across the eye to pass behind and then through the upper iris (Fig. 4.57h). Guide the needle through the corneal incision, taking care not to catch the Descemet's membrane as this is done. The needle is pulled through the superior corneal wound and laid to the side. You can use the Rycroft cannula to guide the tip through the iris (Fig. 4.57i).

(14) The procedure is repeated with the other needle. Leave a gap of approximately 2 mm between the iris punctures.

(15) Pull the upper threads to draw the upper pole of the lens forwards.

(16) Cut off the needles and make the first throw in the suture, and then gently tighten the threads. Check the position of the lens and if happy with its placing and stability, complete the operation.

(17) Complete the upper knot with a triple/single/double sequence.

(18) Complete the lower knot in the same way (Fig. 4.57j).

(19) Cut both knots with long Ong's scissors.

(20) Close the superior corneal wound with a 10-0 nylon suture (Fig. 4.57k). The stab wound is usually self-sealing.

Iris-suturing of IOLs may be combined with closure of existing iris defects (Fig. 4.58). As the knot is pulled tight make sure the haptic lies behind the iris (Fig. 4.59).

When implantation is done during open-sky surgery, the iris suturing is easily accomplished and without the difficult suturing described above. Use 10-0 Prolene sutures mounted on microvascular needles (this will avoid lacerating the iris with spatulated or other needles designed for passing through the sclera and cornea).

SCLERAL FIXATION OF INTRAOCULAR LENSES

Scleral suturing of lenses offers the only chance to implant an intraocular lens in an eye that has suffered devastating damage with loss of iris and all lens remnants. The same technique can be adopted for less extreme circumstances and can even be applied to simple aphakia. The surgery is complicated and technically demanding and requires a careful anterior vitrectomy, possibly with endoscopic visualization. The sutures pass through all the coats of the eye and may provide a route for infection. Positioning the suture so that they only pass through the ciliary sulcus is difficult to censure and recent ultrasound biomicroscopy studies found that only 37 per cent of haptics were adequately located in the ciliary sulcus, but that 48 per cent had vitreous incarceration in the sutured haptics. The difficulties of precisely suturing at the ciliary sulcus, the associated difficulties of iris chafe, pigment dispersion, vitreous incarceration and chronic inflammation mean that there are still problems with this technique. These shortcomings must be remembered when planning surgery, but in any severely damaged eye, IOL implantation (into any position) is rarely going to be 'ideal', and the deficiencies of any technique may well be acceptable when balanced against the handicaps of aphakia.

TECHNIQUE OF PC IOL IMPLANTATION WITH TRANS-SCLERAL SUTURE FIXATION

Choose an IOL with loops built into the haptics, but if such a lens is not available, a 13.5 mm one-piece PMMA lens can be used with sutures tied to the haptics. The lens is usually implanted along an oblique axis to avoid damaging the long ciliary vessels and to respect any future (or

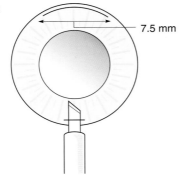

a

7.5 mm

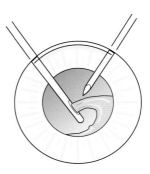

b

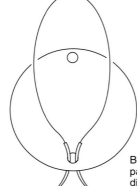

c

Both needles are
passed through the
dialling hole

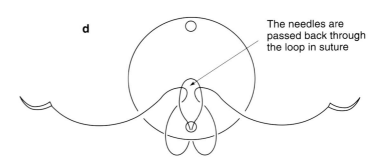

d

The needles are
passed back through
the loop in suture

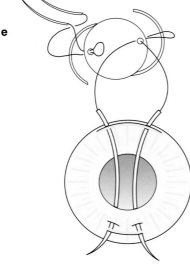

e

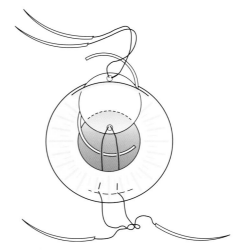

f

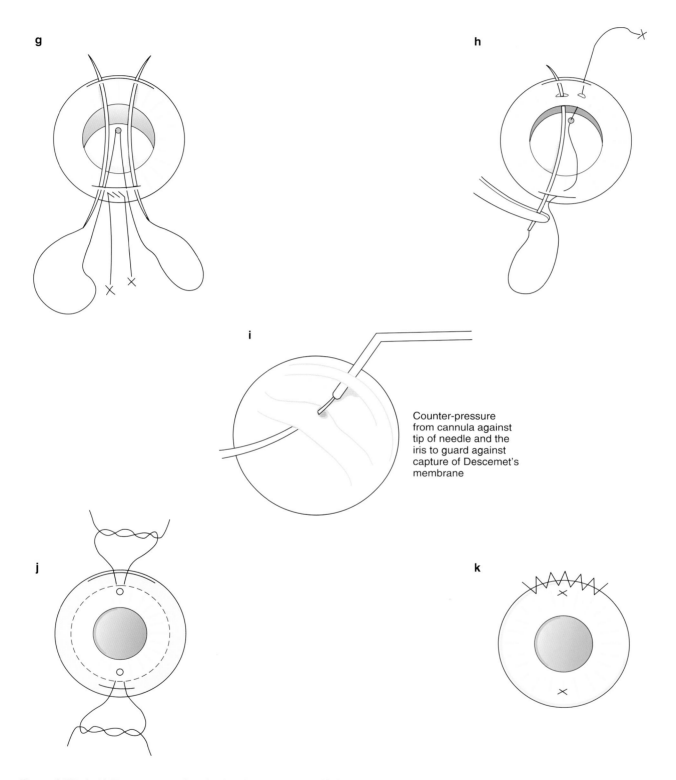

g

h

i

Counter-pressure
from cannula against
tip of needle and the
iris to guard against
capture of Descemet's
membrane

j

k

Figure 4.57. (a–k) The technique of iris fixation; long needles on 10-0 Prolene are tied through the dialling holes on the optic and passed across the anterior chamber, through the mid-periphery of the iris and tied. The process is repeated with another pair of needles, but this time the needles are first passed back to front and then back through the superior, mid-periphery of the iris. The knots are tightened and completed when the IOL is snugly positioned.

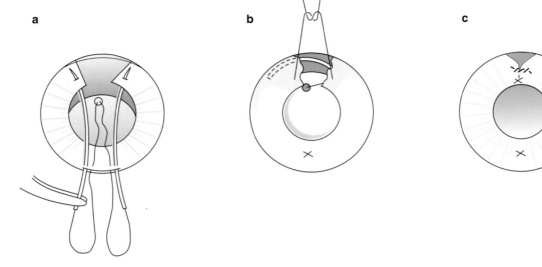

Figure 4.58. (a–c) An iris defect can be closed when performing an iris-sutured IOL implant. Pass the long needles through each pillar of iris and complete the knot; additional sutures may be placed to improve the repair.

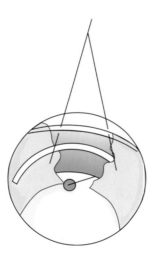

Figure 4.59. Drawing showing a potential hazard when attempting to close an iris defect as part of the operation. If the trailing haptic is lost from sight as the iris is closed, it may come forward into the angle, only to be found there later, on gonioscopy. Make sure this haptic is carefully placed behind the iris.

present) trabeculectomy site. The knots in the supporting sutures must be either rotated into the eye or buried under the scleral flaps.

Preferred sutures: Ethicon 10-0 Prolene, Micropoint plus 16 mm.
Preferred lens: Alcon CZ 70 BD, Pharmacia-UpJohn 722Y.
Alternative lens: Alcon CVC1U, Stortz, Bausch and Lomb 68UV.

There are several ways of suturing a lens to the sclera. The aim is to secure the haptics of an IOL into the ciliary sulcus by sutures passed through the sclera. Whether open-sky or semi-closed, the techniques will vary depending on the lenses and sutures available.

Preparation

A decision to use this technique of implantation must be made before commencing surgery. The technique involves much more manipulation of the globe and is not a 'fall-back' method. Once the eye has been opened and becomes soft, it is difficult to create adequate lamellar flaps or tunnels for trans-scleral suturing.

SINGLE SUTURE TECHNIQUE

(1) Place both superior and inferior rectus sutures using 4-0 Prolene.

(2) Reflect conjunctival flaps in the quadrants chosen for the sutures (usually upper nasal/inferior temporal) and gently cauterize any bleeding points.

(3) Cut two partial thickness radial incisions into the sclera in these oblique meridians. Using a crescent blade, make two pockets at 2 o'clock and 8 o'clock, 180 degrees diametrically opposite each other (Fig. 4.60a).

(4) Make a 7.5 mm partial thickness corneal groove incision, centred on the 12 o'clock position. (It must be 10 mm or larger if implanting a Morcher lens – see earlier.) The lens must be able to pass easily into the eye as the sutures are all pulled up tight.

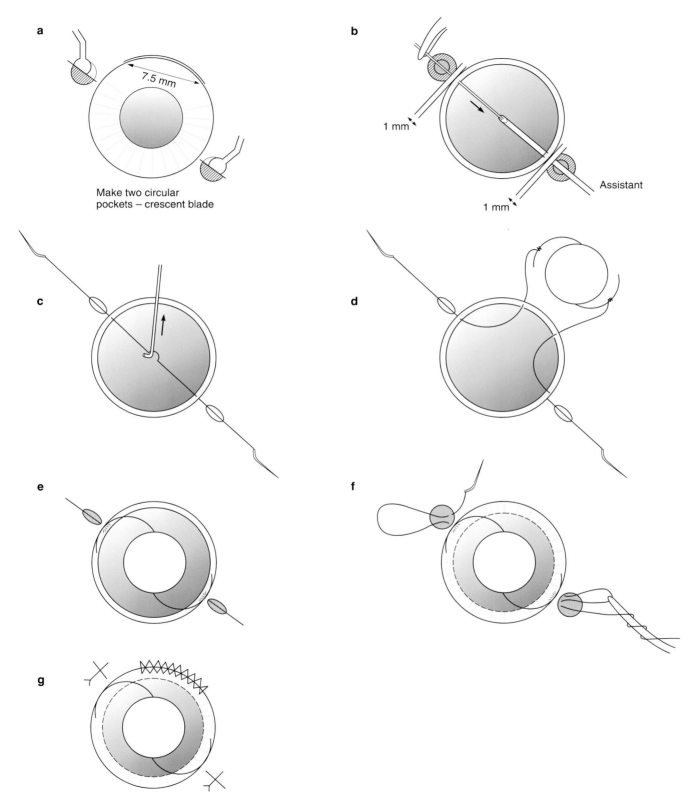

a

7.5 mm

Make two circular
pockets – crescent blade

b

1 mm

1 mm

Assistant

c

d

e

f

g

Figure 4.60. (a–g) Technique for single suture trans-scleral fixation of a PC IOL.

(5) Using stab incisions at either end of this groove, undertake an anterior vitrectomy, indenting the eye to ensure that all vitreous in the region of the ciliary sulcus is removed.

(6) Moisten and apply a self-adhesive Merocel sponge pad to the forehead above the eye (as with iris fixation above). This allows easy manipulation of the lens whilst attaching sutures to it.

(7) Carefully bend a fine hypodermic needle (27-gauge) with Castroviejo needle holders and pass this from outside to in, through the bed of the scleral flap, approximately 1 mm from the limbus. Watch carefully for the tip to appear in the pupil. When the tip is in clear sight, the assistant is given the hypodermic needle to hold in view in the centre of the pupil.

(8) Pass the long needle through the bed of the scleral wound and dock this into the lumen of the hypodermic in the pupil (Fig. 4.60b). Withdraw the hypodermic needle carefully, pushing gently on the needle. When the long needle is clear of the eye, it will easily disengage from the hypodermic and it can be pulled carefully out of the eye with a needle holder.

(9) The suture now spans the eye with a needle at either end. Complete the incision using a diamond knife, cutting from the inside to out, creating a bevelled self-sealing wound. Catch the 10-0 Prolene in the anterior chamber with a Sinskey hook and pull it out of the wound (Fig. 4.60c).

(10) Cut the loop and tie each free end onto the apex of the haptics of the IOL (Fig. 4.60d).

(11) The lens is grasped with McPhearson's forceps and gently posted into the eye as the sutures are pulled up evenly and gently (Fig. 4.60e). Make sure that the lens does not become entangled in the sutures.

(12) The lens should now lie across the posterior chamber supported by the sutures.

(13) Bend the needle and pass it through the bed of the scleral flap dissection and then tie the suture onto itself (Fig. 4.60f). Before completing the knot, check carefully the tightness of the suture and the position of the lens. Remember that the eye will have become very soft after both the anterior vitrectomy and the manipulation and it is possible to over-tighten the suture. Complete the knot with two, then three throws and cut the suture.

(14) Bury the ends under the flap or in the pocket (Fig. 4.60g). Suture the flat to the sclera with 10-0 nylon or 8-0 Dexon.

(15) Complete any other surgical tasks such as iris repair and then close the cornea with 10-0 nylon.

(16) Close the scleral flaps with 10-0 nylon and the conjunctiva with 8-0 or 10-0 vicryl.

(17) Reinflate the eye with balanced salt solution and check for water tightness.

ALTERNATIVE TECHNIQUE

There are alternative ways of suturing to the lens. If the available lens has eyelets on the haptics, use a double-armed suture and the technique below:

(1) Make two scleral pockets, either at 8 o'clock and 2 o'clock or at 4 o'clock and 10 o'clock.

(2) Create a 7.5 mm partial thickness limbal groove. Pass one of the needles into the eye, through the floor of the scleral pocket, 1 mm from the limbus to emerge behind the iris.

(3) As before, dock the tip of this needle into a 27-gauge hypodermic needle which has previously pierced the sclera at the opposite pocket. Pass another needle in the same way 2 mm apart from the first puncture (Fig. 4.61a). Alternatively, pass the same needle back, passing through the floor of the scleral pocket 2 mm from where it initially emerged. Dock the tip in a hypodermic as before and bring it out the other site.

(4) Complete the corneal incision. Use a Sinskey hook to pull each thread out separately; cut off the needles and pass the suture through the loop on the haptic, tying the ends together (Fig. 4.61b). The thread should now run freely through the loop.

(5) Implant the IOL into the eye behind the iris, making sure that the sutures do not entangle the haptics.

(6) Pull the thread back and forth until it runs freely and the knot is out of the eye (Fig. 4.61c). Cut off the excess thread, including the previous knot.

(7) Tie the two ends together and rotate the new knot so that it lies within the eye (Fig. 4.61d). The suture will be covered by the self-sealing scleral pocket. Suture the pocket if necessary.

TRANS-SCLERAL FIXATION DURING CORNEAL GRAFTING

The technique can be used in combination with a penetrating keratoplasty.

Technique

Sutures: Ethicon TG 14D, 10-0 Prolene, double-armed.

(1) Before making the trephine, make two scleral pockets for the sutures (Fig. 4.62a).

(2) Use a trephine sufficiently large to admit the IOL; 8 mm will be the minimum for a Morcher opaque haptic IOL.

(3) Tie the suture to the apex curve of the haptics of the lens or pass through the hoops on the haptics (Fig. 4.62b). Pass each needle in turn behind the iris, through the ciliary sulcus, aiming to penetrate the

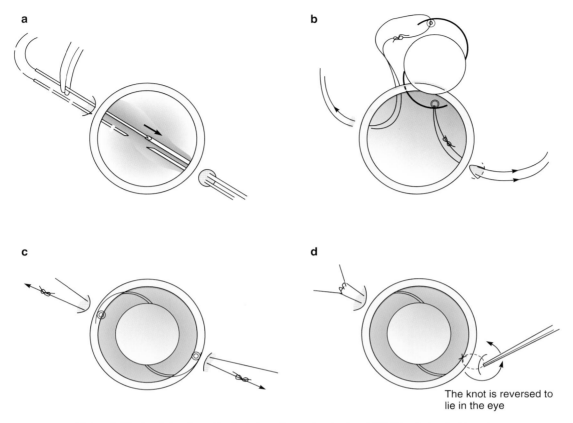

a

b

c

d

The knot is reversed to lie in the eye

Figure 4.61. (a–d) An alternative technique for a scleral-sutured PC IOL using a double suture.

sclera, approximately 1 mm from the limbus, in the bed of one or two scleral pockets (Fig. 4.62b). Pass the two needles so that they emerge approximately 1–2 mm apart.

(4) Repeat for the opposite hole of the lens.

(5) Draw the suture up steadily, then pass the lens through the pupil holding onto both haptics with either plain or McPhearson's forceps (Fig. 4.62c).

(6) Draw the sutures up tight. Ensure they do not catch around the lens as the suture is drawn up.

(7) Cut off the needles and for each knot complete with a 3, 1, 3 pattern of throws (Fig. 4.62d).

(8) Complete the corneal graft.

WOUND CLOSURE

A well-constructed section should be complemented by accurate stitching to close it. Every wound must be water-tight. Use a suturing technique that will allow the closure of the eye rapidly and adjustment as it is inflated to normal IOP. After all the manipulations, interrupted stitches tend to leak and continuous suturing gives better closure;

running as a bootlace from middle to end and then across and back to the middle for the final knot to be tied.

Technique (see Figs 4.63a–e)

The suture is started in the middle of the wound, making the first pass on the deep surface. In a series of generous bites, move to one end and then back to the other end before returning to the middle of the wound where the knot is to be tied. Tension on this stitch can be increased whilst testing until it is water-tight. The knot can then be completed in the depths of the wound. If, as the stitch is tightened, viscoelastic needs to be aspirated or further manipulations are required, the suture can be eased and the anterior chamber re-entered or aspirated.

Corneal grafting

After corneal grafting, it is crucial that the sutures remain quietly in place for at least 1 year; this is the usual minimum time taken for healing to be sufficient for all sutures to be removed. The graft must not leak either at the end of the surgery or at any later date. Loose sutures threaten graft

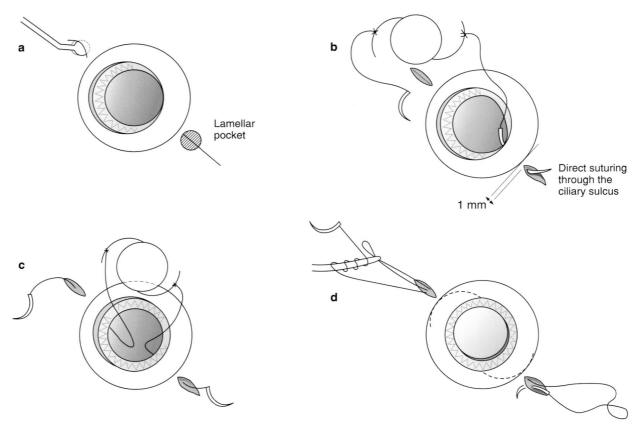

Figure 4.62. (a–d) Direct transcleral suturing through the ciliary sulcus for scleral fixation of IOL during corneal grafting.

survival and accelerate graft rejection, threatening infection of the suture tracks, or breakdown of the graft–host interface with unacceptable levels of induced astigmatism as the donor button slides forward on the host tissue. There are four ways to suture a corneal graft:

(1) Continuous suture.
(2) Interrupted sutures.
(3) Combination of interrupted and continuous sutures.
(4) Double continuous sutures.

For any eye with focal disease, or associated with severe inflammation, interrupted stitching is the safest. There is a risk of the sutures becoming loose if the disease recurs in the graft and, if a continuous stitch has been used, the whole of this would become loose. Combined (continuous and interrupted) does give the added control of being able to remove sutures to correct astigmatism as the eye begins to heal; suture removal is done in the axis of the plus cylinder.

Always pass the needle into strong tissue, extending the passage of the tip of the needle until such tissue is reached. If the suture track passes beyond the peripheral cornea into the conjunctiva, it will be difficult to tighten the suture; to avoid this, pull the conjunctiva tight as the needle pierces it.

Closure of small wounds

The small wounds used for second instruments, or self-retaining infusions often leak after extended manipulation. Closure is ensured with either a single radial or a mattress suture. Make sure the knots are buried. Start the mattress on the deep surface and tie the knot in the depths of the wound.

Joining sutures together

There are several circumstances when it may be necessary to tie one fine suture to another, e.g. if a 10-0 nylon stitch breaks during a corneal graft; when scleral suturing an IOL; when a knot is needed to re-join the cut ends a stitch; to tie a different needle to the end of a suture, to do a scleral bite. The simplest way to do this is to use a fishing knot called the 'dropper knot'. This is an invaluable trick for any microsurgeon.

TECHNIQUE

Take the two ends that are to be tied together and align them so that the ends lie side by side. Bend them together in a

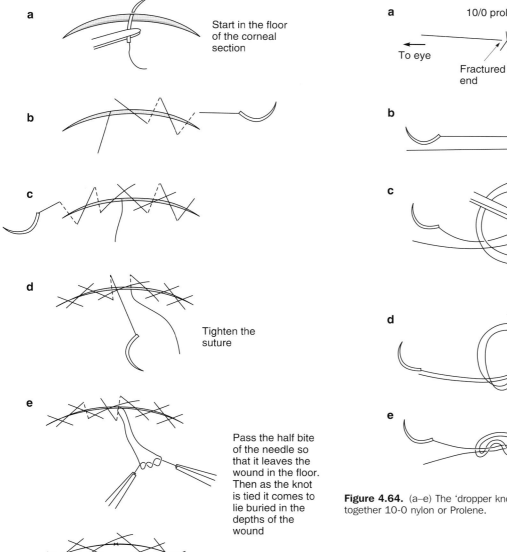

a Start in the floor of the corneal section

b

c

d Tighten the suture

e Pass the half bite of the needle so that it leaves the wound in the floor. Then as the knot is tied it comes to lie buried in the depths of the wound

Figure 4.63. (a–e) Simple continuous suture for closing corneal incisions.

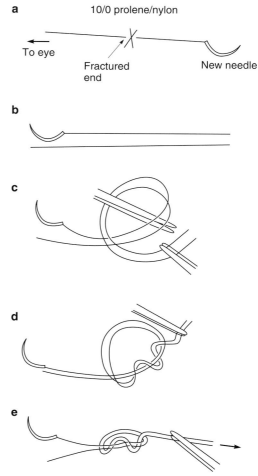

a 10/0 prolene/nylon
To eye
Fractured end
New needle

b

c

d

e

Figure 4.64. (a–e) The 'dropper knot', an easy way of joining together 10-0 nylon or Prolene.

generous loop, and with micro tying forceps and a pair of McPhearson's, twist the thread two or three times around the loop. Pulling on both, tighten the knot. Leave some excess suture so that the knot will not undo as it is pulled through cornea or sclera. It takes a little practice, but is sound. The track made by the needle is sufficiently large to allow the new knot to easily pass (see Figs 4.64a–e).

All knots should be buried and the ends tucked into the wound to avoid post-operative discomfort. Use interrupted stitches if the wounds leak after suturing.

The McCannel stitch is one of the fundamental knots of advanced microsurgery. Its use for closing iris defects has already been described above, but it can also be used to

help capture the haptics of displacing lenses and indeed its early uses were particularly to help stabilize iris clip lenses that were threatening to dislocate (Fig. 4.65).

SQUINT SURGERY

In any patient where there has been a delay between insult and reconstruction, fusion may have been lost, and as a result the eye becomes divergent. Correction of the ocular position in these patients poses the added risk of intractable diplopia, but this is rarely (but not never) found in practice. The patient must be warned that a good result in terms of a return of vision may accentuate the clarity of the images but produce diplopia. Orthoptic assessment may help, but in reality, if the vision is too poor to give useful responses on functional testing, counselling and

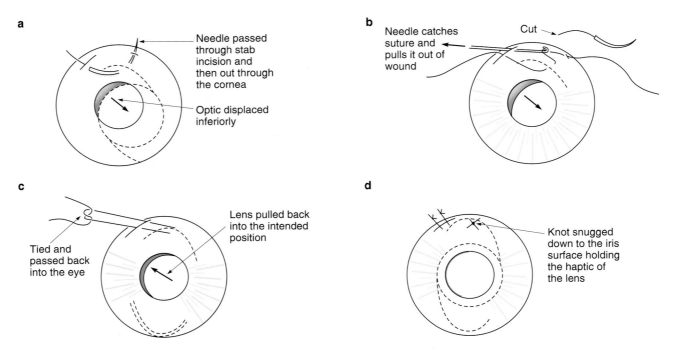

a

Needle passed through stab incision and then out through the cornea

Optic displaced inferiorly

b

Needle catches suture and pulls it out of wound

Cut

c

Lens pulled back into the intended position

Tied and passed back into the eye

d

Knot snugged down to the iris surface holding the haptic of the lens

Figure 4.65. (a–d) Drawings showing use of the McCannel suture to recapture the haptic of an IOL sinking into the vitreous.

support may be all that can be offered. If there is a large angle of deviation, an injection of botulinum toxin into the appropriate muscle (e.g. into the lateral rectus, if the eye is divergent), given at the end of reconstructive surgery, can usually produce an improvement of position and even return of fusion. Adjustable muscle surgery may also be tried, but as a delayed operation. This should be done by a strabismologist and after the eye has had a chance to recover as much vision as possible. However, because the problems and possibility of diplopia remain, surgery on the ocular muscles may achieve no more than cosmetic improvement.

Chapter 5

Management of post-operative problems

INTRODUCTION

The post-operative course following reconstruction may be complicated. Particular problems with haemorrhage, glaucoma and corneal oedema can be expected if the primary insult or surgery was complicated. The immediate post-operative period needs careful supervision and an appropriately energetic response when problems occur. It is important to have warned the patient of possible post-operative problems, reminding them that the outcomes are clearly less predictable than those from primary elective surgery. Having said that, the post-operative course is usually unremarkable and preparation of the eye before surgery, and the surgical removal of any irritating factors such as a loose IOL, should have alleviated most of the pre-operative problems.

ROUTINE POST-OPERATIVE MANAGEMENT

The patient is examined on the first day and treatment is titrated against the physical signs of inflammatory activity and intraocular pressure. The routine followed is presented in Table 5.1, and a suggested post-operative regimen of medication is presented in Table 5.2.

The patients are usually discharged home the day after surgery but can be managed as day cases. Most importantly, they must be able to attend frequently if the post-operative course turns out to be complicated. They are next reviewed at one week and then at less frequent intervals as the eye recovers. By the end of the first week the eye should be very much less inflamed and the frequency of topical medication reduced appropriately – down to once or twice a day by one month. The antibiotics can usually be

Table 5.1. Day one post-operative examination.

History	
Complaints	Ask about symptoms of pain, discomfort or blurring. Some degree of all three should be expected.
Examination	
Visual acuity	This should be documented unaided, with glasses or with a pin-hole. If it is below 6/60, check for an afferent pupil defect and light projection.
Possible findings:	
Conjunctiva	Injection, haemorrhage.
Wound	Check that the wound is water-tight and that all knots are buried.
Cornea	Fine oedema may be seen close to the wound, especially if the surgical manipulations were prolonged. The presence of corneal oedema may indicate that IOP is raised.
Anterior chamber	Residual viscoelastic, haemorrhage, inflammatory cells, flare and fibrin will be seen but should settle within a week. Fibrin will be prominent if there has been extensive iris manipulation.
Intraocular pressure	Applanation is not always easy on the first post-operative day but IOP should be checked.
Retina	Check for a red reflex which should be visible, although retinal details may not easily be seen until corneal clarity returns and any haemorrhage or other debris have cleared from the AC.

Table 5.2. Post-operative treatment.

Topical steroids	Gutt. Prednisolone acetate 1 per cent , two hourly for four days, then reducing to four times per day
Topical antibiotics	Gutt. Chloramphenicol, four times a day for two weeks
Hypotensives	Small doses of acetozolamide in divided doses (e.g. 125 mg 3x daily, Diamox Slow Release 250 mg twice daily) may be used in the immediate post-operative period to control any rise in IOP. In a grafted eye, where IOP measurements are difficult to obtain immediately after surgery, acetazolamide can be given if there is any corneal oedema.
Discharge	Patients are usually discharged home the day after surgery but can be managed as day cases. They must be able to attend for frequent out-patient examinations if the post-operative course turns out to be complicated.

stopped after two weeks, and systemic acetozolamide is discontinued when the IOP is normal.

Patients can be refracted for the first time at about eight weeks. Glasses can be prescribed at this early stage if the prescription is tolerable, but the sutures should not be removed before 12 weeks from the operation, particularly if a continuous suture has been used to close the wound. Extend this time if steroid treatment has been excessive.

Any sudden changes in vision should be immediately reported and the patient examined to find the cause. Retinal detachment, cystoid macula oedema, corneal decompensation and glaucoma can, among other problems, cause a change in vision.

The patient is normally reviewed monthly until it is clear that all is progressing well and then the intervals may be extended considerably. After one year it is our practice to review all these patients annually. Some eyes will not settle so easily, and daily, dilute steroid drops will be needed on a protracted basis to keep the eye quiet and prevent inflammatory cells depositing on the IOL. Long-term follow-up will be needed for any eye exhibiting such chronic inflammation. If a corneal graft was needed, the follow-up will necessarily be more intense and extended. The visual return in these eyes will be slower and topical steroids may be needed for much longer, sometimes for several years.

SPECIFIC COMPLICATIONS

Specific problems include:

(1) Inflammation.
(2) Intraocular pressure (IOP).
(3) Refraction.
(4) IOL difficulties.
(5) Photophobia.
(6) Squints and diplopia.
(7) Infection.
(8) Problems with corneal grafts.

(1) Inflammation

Inflammation should lessen in the days and weeks following surgery; the frequency and strength of topical steroids are reduced in parallel. However it must be noted that a mild, chronic inflammation often tends to remain, particularly if there had been significant inflammation at the time of presentation. Systemic steroids are rarely if ever required to treat these patients.

Any pre-operative uveitis should be treated with steroids during the weeks before surgery. After the operation, the inflammatory response may be brisk, with profuse fibrin formation and a marked cellular response (Fig. 5.1). In these circumstances, strong steroid drops, e.g. prednisolone 1 per cent forte, given frequently, will contain the inflammation within a week or two. Alternative causes such as infection must also always be considered if the uveitis is sustained in spite of this intensive regimen.

In those eyes which have suffered surgical insults to the iris, it is not uncommon to notice fine flare and an occasional cell in the anterior chamber, indicating established damage to the iris and a chronically leaky blood–eye barrier. This inflammation does not require treatment unless it seems to be increasing.

Sometimes cellular deposits will form on either the IOL or the cornea (as keratic precipitates), reducing vision. A short course of topical steroids will usually clear the cells, but the need for steroids may be sustained for many months. The neodymuim:yttrium, aluminium, garnet (Nd.YAG) laser can destroy these deposits, but although the treatment is effective in the short term, the deposits tend to recur unless also treated with topical steroids (Figs 5.2a and b).

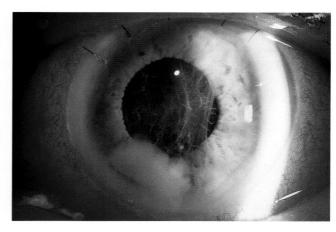

Figure 5.1. Brisk fibrinous uveitis.

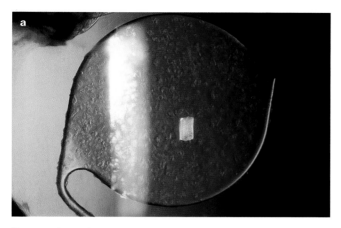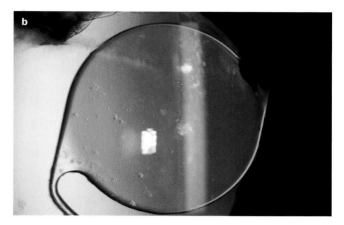

Figure 5.2. (a) Confluent cellular deposits on the IOL after anterior segment reconstruction, reducing vision from 6/6 to 6/36. (b) After two weeks' treatment with topical betamethasone, four times daily, the vision improved, as did the clinical appearance. The reduction in the cellular deposits is obvious and was sustained by daily applications for six months.

Always examine both eyes and be aware that the later development of uveitis in the fellow eye may herald the onset of sympathetic ophthalmia.

Uveitis found in an eye which has had a corneal graft may herald the onset of an acute rejection. An increase in the frequency or potency of the topical steroids is needed and titrated against the response.

(2) Intraocular pressure

Intraocular pressure problems are caused by imbalances between aqueous production and outflow/drainage. Damage to the anterior segment affects not only the optical pathways – the cornea, lens, iris, pupil and vitreous – but also the tissues that control the production and egress of aqueous from the eye. The angle may have been obstructed by vitreous or blocked by adhesions from an incarcerated IOL; pigment shedding will reduce the outflow through the trabecular meshwork; conjunctival scarring will reduce the surgical options and trabecular damage will reduce the effectiveness of drugs needed to control the IOP. Similarly, damage to or detachment of the ciliary body will reduce aqueous production, and threaten hypotony.

The clinical scenario will be determined by which of these variables predominates (see Table 5.3).

RAISED IOP

Raised IOP should be suspected if there is fine corneal oedema (Fig. 5.3) and can be managed in a number of ways:

(a) Systemic acetazolamide.
(b) Topical medication, used singly or in combination.
(c) Trabeculectomy.

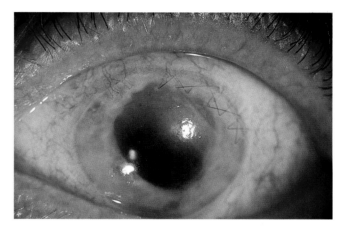

Figure 5.3. Fine corneal oedema following removal of a traumatic cataract.

(d) Augmented trabeculectomy – 5 FU, Mitomicin C.
(e) Tubal implant – Ahmed valve, Molteno tube.
(f) Diode laser.

A transient rise in the IOP is common in the hours or days following anterior segment reconstruction. Any damage to the trabecular meshwork will restrict the egress of blood, fibrin and viscoelastic and this in turn will reduce the flow of aqueous. The pressure rise should be anticipated, and it is therefore routine to give the patient an intravenous injection of acetazolamide (Diamox 250–500 mg) at the end of the operation. This is continued as oral acetazolamide in moderate dosages (Diamox SR 250 mg twice daily; Diamox 125 mg, three times daily) for up to 10 days, if the IOP remains elevated. If the rise is sustained in spite of oral treatment, beta-blocker drops such as Betagan and Timoptol may be added. Usually such medical treatment is adequate.

If there are signs of optic disc damage, surgery must be considered to control the IOP. Although a trabeculectomy would normally be the operation of choice, previous conjunctival inflammation and scarring may predicate against success. An augmented trabeculectomy, using either 5-fluoro-uracil or mitomycin-C should then be considered. Raised IOP threatens the survival of any corneal graft and drainage surgery must be considered at an early stage for these eyes.

Other surgical options include tubal implants (Ahmed valves and Molteno tubes) and diode laser. Tubal implants are not without problems, and their use is better restricted to a glaucoma specialist.

The diode laser on the other hand is easily used and the protocol simple (Figs. 5.4a and b). The laser destroys the ciliary processes and thus reduces the formation of the aqueous.

TECHNIQUE OF DIODE ABLATION OF THE CILIARY BODY EPITHELIUM

Use either a sub-Tenon's or peribulbar local anaesthetic.

A light pipe is used to identify the position of the ciliary body. Perform a series of applicatons around the limbus, directing the tip of the probe at the ciliary body. Treat approximately 270 degrees at the first treatment with 20–30 applications (power 1750 mW; 1.5–2 s duration).

Treatment can be dosed and repeated if the response is inadequate or if the pressure rises again. It is a dramatically effective alternative modality for controlling the IOP in these complicated eyes. Indications include uncontrolled IOP when alternative medications have failed; when surgery is the only option, but when the outcome of such surgery is likely to fail because of local problems such as dense scarring of the conjunctiva, or if previous surgery has failed. Hypotony has been reported, but tends to occur if treatment is too aggressive or if the ciliary body has been partially destroyed by injury. The real advantage is that the treatment may be dosed, one treatment following the other and a few weeks are given to assess the response.

There is a fine line between glaucoma and hypotony in some of these damaged eyes. A typically problematical presentation is the eye of a 15-year-old male patient who had an intense cyclitis after a penetrating injury. All settled

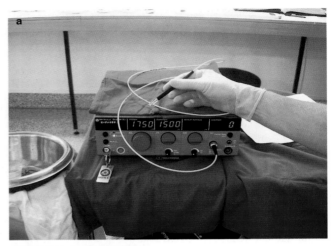

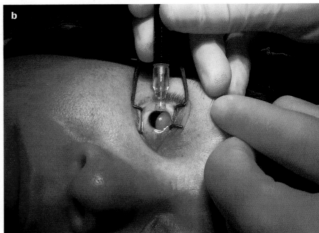

Figure 5.4. (a) The diode laser (Iris Medical) showing typical settings. (b) The diode probe is applied directly to the eye under local anaesthetic.

and the patient underwent a sulcus-fixated secondary lens implant. He developed high IOP of 37 mmHg some eight months after surgery. The initially successful response to a beta-blocker suddenly faded, and the IOP rose to a point where acetazolamide was needed. This controlled the IOP for four weeks and he then presented, via the accident and

Table 5.3. IOP problems following reconstructive surgery.

Situation	Aqueous production	Aqueous drainage	IOP	Response to medication	Next step
Routine	Normal	Normal	Normal	None	
Open angle glaucoma	Raised Normal	Normal Reduced	Raised Raised	Beta-blockers Diamox	
Cyclodialysis	Reduced	Increased	Hypotony	None	Cyclopexy
Damaged ciliary body	Reduced	Reduced	Raised or low		
Damaged angle	Normal	Reduced	Raised	Little or none	Diode laser

emergency department, with poor vision. On examination, the IOP was noted to be 6 mmHg and stayed down at this level for some weeks despite withdrawal of treatment. Then, some three weeks later, the patient presented again with poor vision and an IOP of 45 mmHg. The cycle was repeated. The dose of acetazolamide was halved and the IOP stabilized and has remained satisfactory for the next five years.

A possible reason for this fragility of pressure control is damage to both outflow pathways and the ciliary body. In this circumstance, if a trabeculectomy is performed to 'control' IOP, the eye may remain soft because there is insufficient ciliary body to produce sufficient aqueous to overcome the new 'improved' outflow. The IOP will be persistently low with the associated problems of hypotony (choroidal folds, disc and macular oedema and suprachoroidal haemorrhages). The end-result of this process will be phthisis bulbi.

Once the possible causes of the observed fluctuations in post-operative pressure are understood, it becomes easier to manage them more effectively. If damage to both outflow and production pathways is suspected, lower doses of oral acetazolamide, 125 mg two or three times a day, should be tried as a first line treatment and tapered off as indicated. Beta-blockers and other drops can be introduced if the IOP is persistently high, but with care unless the IOP crashes.

HYPOTONY

If the IOP is consistently low, the possibility that the surgical manipulations have aggravated or caused a disinsertion of the ciliary body must be remembered. For instance, the attempt to suture an IOL into the ciliary sulcus can cause a ciliary body haemorrhage or disinsertion of this tiny piece of tissue. Gonioscopy should establish whether there is disinsertion or not. Complete disinsertion is recognized by a cyclodialysis cleft (Fig. 5.5). The management of these clefts depends on their extent and their effects on the eye. If the IOP is moderate (approximately 10 mmHg) and the cleft is small, it can often be managed conservatively, i.e. given time and topical steroid drops. Small clefts can be closed using argon laser trabeculoplasty or cyclo-cryotherapy.

Surgical repair of the cleft (cyclopexy) should be considered if the hypotony persists. In this circumstance, the cleft will usually be extensive, the vision poor and be associated with macular oedema, choroidal folds or both. The IOP

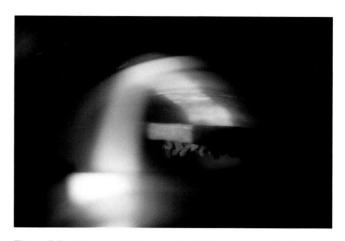

Figure 5.5. A huge cyclodialysis cleft with iris root and ciliary body stretched out like washing to dry. The IOP was 6 mmHg. Chronic retinal changes were also visible.

will often be less than 5 mmHg. The technique is described in Figs 5.6a–e.

(3) Refraction

At eight weeks, with a wound of 7.5 mm, the eye should be stable enough to order a preliminary refraction. This should be done within a couple of weeks in children, to give the child the best possible vision and prevent amblyopia. At the very least the glasses will provide a platform for patching and the start of orthoptic rehabilitation (see Chapter 6).

All sutures, including any tight stitches causing with-the-rule (WTR) astigmatism, should be left in place for about 12 weeks before removal. Secondary wounds take longer to regain pre-operative strength. With a row of interrupted sutures, it is better to remove individual sutures one at a time. If the sutures are removed too soon the wound will tend to sag causing against-the-rule (ATR) astigmatism.

The majority of pre-presbyopic patients will prefer a distance-only correction for their 'new' eye. They will continue to accommodate and read with their undamaged eye. Presbyopic patients can be prescribed multifocal glasses for both eyes (see Table 5.4).

Table 5.4. Prescribing spectacles in patients with unilateral pseudophakia following reconstruction (this will depend on the vision and potential for vision).

Patient group	Undamaged eye	Damaged eye
Child (under 8)	Bifocal (+1.00 add)	Bifocal (+2.25 add). Contact lens for distance with reading correction
Teenager/pre-presbyopic	Distance only	Distance only
Presbyopes	Bifocal or varifocal	Bifocal or varifocal

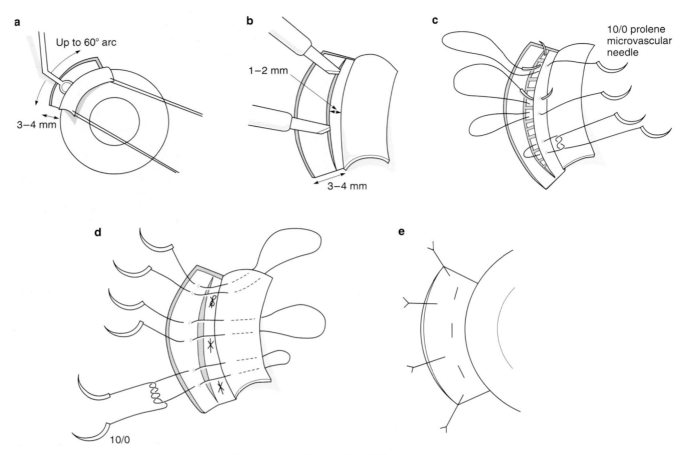

Figure 5.6. (a–e) The technique of cyclopexy (after Demeler). (See also Fig. 2.9.)

If there is a reasonable similarity in the refraction of the two eyes, and the acuity is good, patients will often accept the full correction. The patient should be encouraged to wear their glasses constantly in the hope of restoring or maintaining fusion. If there is marked or irregular astigmatism or an anisometopia of greater than 3 dioptres other refractive options may be tried (Fig. 5.7).

ASTIGMATISM

Regular astigmatism is usually caused by wounds in the corneal periphery. Astigmatism may be WTR, plus axis between 70 and 110 degrees, usually caused by tight sutures, or ATR, plus axis at, or around 180 degrees, which is usually caused by wound collapse or loose sutures.

The treatment of post-operative astigmatism will depend on its degree, axis and whether sutures remain in place or not. Ideally, at the end of the operation, the eye should have between 1 and 3 dioptres of WTR astigmatism, most, or all, induced by the sutures. When the sutures are removed the WTR astigmatism should reduce or dis-

appear, but may become ATR if the tissues are weak, or if the suture line has been inflamed.

Mild to moderate (2.5 dioptres or less) astigmatism can be managed with spectacles but if greater than 2.5–3 diop-

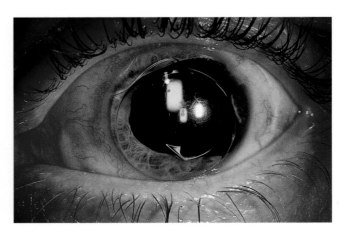

Figure 5.7. This pseudophakic patient wears a contact lens to treat the irregular astigmatism of his scarred cornea.

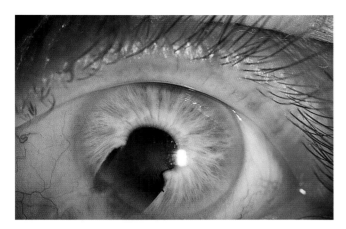

Figure 5.14. Limbal wound, lens collapse and a 'key-hole' pupil.

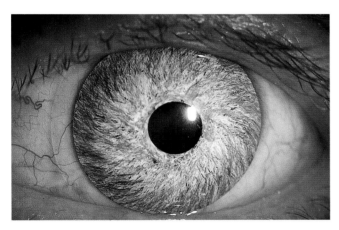

Figure 5.15. The eye from Fig 5.14 treated with a cosmetic contact lens.

Post-operative diplopia is not usually a problem even if a squint was present before surgery. Some patients, usually those with moderate visual return, are happy to have just had the cosmetic and physical problems relieved. In these patients the squint can be ignored. However, if diplopia persists, it is important to establish what the patient means by 'double' vision. Ghosting and superimposition of images can be caused by edge effects from poorly centred lenses or large unreactive pupils, and aniseikonia will result if there is a marked refractive imbalance. Truly separated images are due to strabismus and this misalignment can be corrected with muscle surgery.

Different surgeons recommend different techniques, but adjustable muscle surgery has the advantage of giving the patient subjective input into the final position of the eye. The patient should be warned that the risks of diplopia increase the closer the visual axes get to each other. Orthoptic involvement is particularly helpful and their input to this stage of rehabilitation may include the prescription of prisms or occlusion.

A squinting eye is as much a cosmetic blemish handicap as an eye with an unsightly corneal scar (Fig. 5.16). If the patient is also suffering from diplopia, the poor functional outcome will compound the social and cosmetic problems.

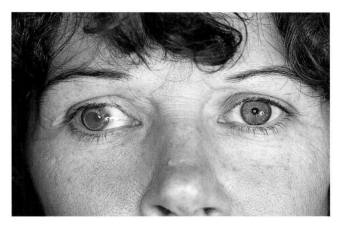

Figure 5.16. The cosmetic and social problems of a divergent squint may be as severe as the visual handicap.

(7) Infection

Post-operative infection remains an intermittent, and fortunately infrequent, complication. This is surprising because by the very nature of reconstructive surgery there are more opportunities for inoculation. The surgery takes longer and involves more steps than routine cataract surgery.

A patient with infective endophthalmitis will present two to four days after surgery, with a history of loss of vision, increasing pain and redness in the eye. The classical signs of inflammation (rapidly increasing cellular and fibrinous effusion, hypopyon and vitritis) will vary in timing and degree according to the virulence of the organism. Examples of an acute fulminating infection, acute endophthalmitis associated with a leaking wound and a chronic capsular abscess are shown in Figs 5.17, 5.18 and 5.19, respectively. In any case where inflammation increases after surgery, the possibility of infection must be considered and appropriate steps taken to identify and treat the organism, sooner rather than later. If it is impossible to see into the posterior segment, an ultrasound will then be required to assess whether the retina or vitreous are detached. A suggested protocol for the management of endophthalmitis is presented in Table 5.6 and Fig. 5.20.

(8) Problems with corneal grafts

The pathological setting of many of these eyes is not ideal for corneal grafting. The integrity of the anterior chamber has previously been breached and chronic inflammation,

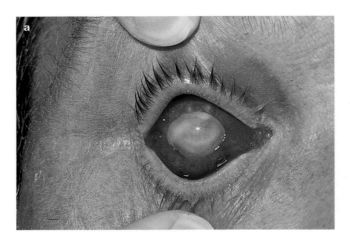
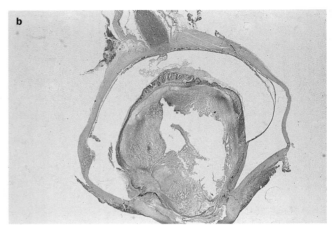

Figure 5.17. (a, b) Acute fulminating endophthalmitis with its corresponding post-enucleation histology.

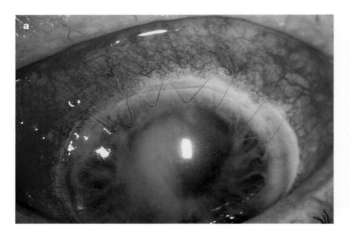
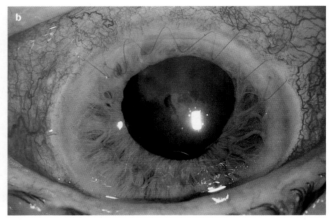

Figure 5.18. (a) Acute post-operative endophthalmitis related to a leaking wound (note the inferior wound which may be associated with infection more frequently). (b) The same eye as (a) a week after intracameral and intravitreal antibiotics. The patient was still on topical and systemic treatment and shows resolution in progress.

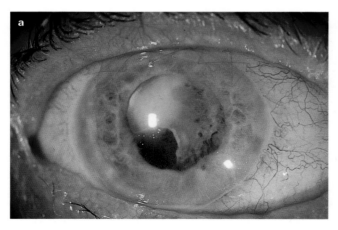
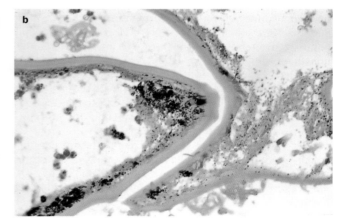

Figure 5.19. (a) Chronic infection with *Staphylococcus epidermidis* leading to a capsular abscess. (b) Histology from the case in (a) showing a fibrinous exudate and heavy bacterial contamination. The IOL was explanted within the capsular bag.

complex pseudophakia, glaucoma, vascularization, both superficial and deep, is a frequent finding.

It is not therefore surprising that the management of any eye which has undergone allograft corneal grafting is detailed, extended and frequently complicated. (The opportunity to do a rotational graft should always be taken.)

The particular problems may be listed as follows:

(a) Optical.
(b) Rejection.
(c) Glaucoma.

OPTICAL

The shape of the host cornea is modified by the injury or previous surgery. Small grafts tend to be most influenced by the shape of the host and will tend to be less stable in terms of their refraction. Larger grafts will have a better shape and less astigmatism, but their increased size brings the graft–host interface closer to the vascular limbus, and this in turn increases immune recognition and rejection, and suture-related problems (e.g. vascularization, loosening).

Excessive astigmatism is approached conservatively and then invasively. Refraction and topographic assessment will identify the trends in the shape of the cornea in the months after surgery. Sutures which are too tight can be removed. They will usually lie at either end of the axis of the plus cylinder. The post-operative steroid requirement will be greater following re- or complex grafts than after routine transplantation; hence the healing of the corneal interface will de delayed. You should wait a minimum of three months from the time of the operation before starting to remove sutures. It is not normally practical to fit contact lenses much before one year post-operatively, and the skill of a specialist fitter is essential. Spectacle over-correction is also useful and frequently used.

After 12 months, and not before because of problems with healing, any significant residual problems with astigmatism require a clear strategic approach. Before offering surgical intervention other than suture removal, all sutures are removed and the remaining astigmatism is considered for treatment. Refraction and topography will help identify areas where corneal shape is most affected and where surgery can be directed. The options include relieving incisions including arcuate keratotomies, Ruiz keratotomies and incisions into the graft–host interface, tension sutures and wedge excision, or combinations of the above. Excimer laser, particularly using LASIK, also has the potential to help these eyes, but the risk is that the refraction will still be changing some years after the graft, and the laser will have to be repeated. It does have the particular benefit that both the cylindrical and spherical components can be treated.

Relaxing incisions in the graft interface can treat 0–10 dioptres of astigmatism. The surgery is simply done but the

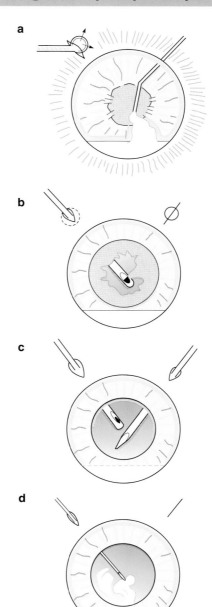

Figure 5.20. (a) Make a scleral pocket with a crescent blade. A paracentesis is used to aspirate the hypopyon. Fill the anterior chamber with viscoelastic. The AC aspirate is sent for analysis. (b) Use an MVR blade to enter the eye through the scleral pocket. Use the tip to open any cyclitic membrane. The vitrector is passed into the centre of the pupil and a specimen of vitreous in this region is removed for analysis. (c) A second scleral pocket can be used to provide access for a separate infusion if a vitrectomy is required. (d) Using the scleral incision, antibiotic is injected into the anterior vitreous. Note that the bevel is turned to face the cornea and that the injection is given slowly.

outcome is unpredictable and seems to induce a period of prolonged instability in the graft. Additional effect can be obtained by placing one or two 10-0 Prolene compression sutures at right angles to the relieving incisions. Depending

Table 5.6. The management of endophthalmitis.

Post-traumatic	Acute post-operative	Chronic post-op
Incidence		
Overall 7%	Cataract 0.07 – 0.13%	Sporadic
Rural pop. up to 30%	Drainage 0.06–1.8%	
Organisms		
S. epidermidis	*Staph.epidermidis (70%)*	*Staph.epidermidis*
Bacillus cereus	*Staph.aureus (10%)*	*Proprionobacter acnes*
Streptococcus spp,	*Streptococcus* spp. *(9%)*	*Candida* spp.
	Gram-negative org. (6%)	
Presentation		
Photophobia	Pain, photophobia	Persistent low-grade uveitis
Intense pain	Discharge, reduced VA	Posterior capsular plaque
Panuveitis	Chemosis, injection	
Hypopyon	Anterior and posterior	
Afferent pupil defect	Uveitis and hypopyon	
Poor vision	Afferent pupil defect	> 6/52 post-surgery
	<1/52 post-surgery	
Risk factors		
Lens disruption, IOFB	Blepharitis, prolonged, surgery, capsular rupture, concomitant respiratory infection	No specific risk factors known
Agricultural injury		
Delayed primary repair		
Diagnosis		
Anterior chamber tap and vitreous biopsy to identify the organism	Ant. chamber tap and vitreous biopsy to identify the organism	Excision-biopsy of the plaque

Treatment

It is important to start antibiotic treatment as quickly as possible. It should be given before the culture results are available. Vancomycin 1 mg/0.1 ml and ceftazidime 2.25 mg/0.1 ml or amikacin 0.4 mg/0.1 ml are the antibiotics of choice for intra-vitreal use. The antibiotics are given in separate syringes.

Post-traumatic	Acute post-operative	Chronic post-op
Outcome		
Poorest outcomes 30% better than 20/400	Depends on organism	Good visual prognosis
	20/100 or better with:	
	S. epidermidis 84%	
	Gram-negative 56%	
	S. aureus 50%	
	Streptococci 30%	
Prophylaxis		
Prompt primary repair	5 per cent povidone-iodine preparation	As for acute endophthalmitis
Early use of antibiotics	Pre-op. topical antibiotics	
Removal of all foreign material		
Recommended treatment dosages		
Intravitreal	Ceftazidime, 2.25 mg in 0.1 ml	
	Vancomycin, 1.0 mg in 0.1 ml	
	Amikacin, 0.4 mg in 0.1 ml	
Subconjunctival	Ceftazidime, 100 mg in 0.5 ml	
	Vancomycin, 25 mg in 0.5ml	
Topical	Ceftazidime, 100 mg/ml drops hourly	
	Vancomycin, 50 mg/ml drops hourly	
Systemic	Ciprofloxacin, 750 mg twice daily OR	
	Ceftazidime, 1g intravenously every 8 hours	
	Vancomycin, 1 g intravenously every 12 hours	
	(both these drugs should be used with caution in patients with renal problems)	
	Prednisolone, 1 mg/kg daily for 5–10 days	

Table 5.6. continued
Acute post-operative endophthalmitis
Early vitrectomy may improve the visual prognosis.

Chronic endophthalmitis
As for acute post-operative endophthalmitis but only using the intra-vitreal and topical treatment routes

Post-traumatic endophthalmitis
Bacillus cereus will produce a fulminating endophthalmitis with signs of systemic involvement including pyrexia. Vancomycin and aminoglycosides have a synergistic benefit against this organism.

Kresloff, M.S., Castellarin, A.A. and Zarbin, M.A. (1998). Endopthalmitis. *Survey of Ophthalmology*, **43**(3), 193–224.

on the outcome, these are removed one at a time, at eight weeks and then at 12 weeks later, but left in place if there has been full correction.

Arcuate cuts can be used in the same way as the relieving incisions. The smaller the optical zone, and the deeper the incisions, the greater will be the effect of the surgery. When relieving keratotomies are combined with radial cuts (Ruiz procedure), a reduction in astigmatism 3–12 dioptres can be corrected. Again, under- and over-correction is possible; however the corneal curvature will tend to be flattened, reducing myopic and increasing hyperopic spherical refraction. The treatment is best used on those eyes which have a myopic spherical equivalent.

Compression sutures can be useful, particularly in the months after surgery when there is obviously flattening in one area of the graft. 10-0 Prolene is used rather than nylon because the suture lasts longer and does not hydrolyse as quickly in ultraviolet light. The tightening effect of these sutures is to increase the curvature of the cornea, increasing the myopia.

Wedge excision is reserved for higher degrees of astigmatism (10–15 dioptres) and is more difficult to do. An arc of cornea is removed with a diamond blade, and the wound sutured with 10-0 Prolene. Approximately 1–2 dioptres of correction is achieved for every 0.1 mm removed. If more than this is removed it is difficult to close the wound and unacceptable steepening of the cornea will result.

GRAFT REJECTION

Rejection and graft failure are constant threats in all these eyes. The risk is higher in those which have glaucoma, or that have continuing background inflammation, e.g. those that had iris damage or needed suturing through vascular tissues to achieve lens implantation. This inflammation must always be contained and suppressed. Long-term topical steroids, used perhaps no more than once a day, may need to be continued for several years. Regular follow-up and open access to the clinics will help identify problems earlier rather than later. Enrolling the patient's co-operation, and teaching them to be aware of symptoms, will improve the chance to treat rejection episodes early.

The signs of rejection are reduced visual acuity, inflammation (Fig. 5.21), with or without classical rejection line formation (Fig. 5.22), and total or regional corneal oedema. If the clinical appearance is unclear, it is better to review

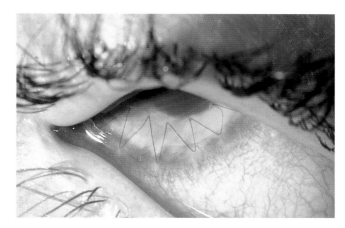

Figure 5.21. Acute graft rejection. A 15-year-old male post-corneal/lens laceration. He presented with pain, photophobia and loss of vision nine months after surgery.

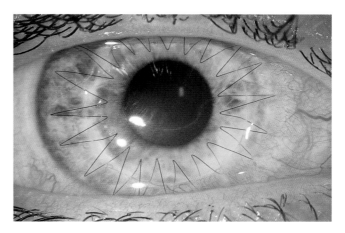

Figure 5.22. Epithelial rejection line. A 57-year-old male was grafted for pseudophakic bullous keratopathy. Three months after surgery he presented with a short history of reduced vision.

the patient a week later. The detection in any graft patient of an increase in inflammation must alert to the possibility of a rejection episode. Superficial vessels growing to or over the interface must be watched, but the growth of deep vessels into the graft–host interface is a serious event and needs a response. The vessels usually grow in relation to sutures, sometimes following their tracks. They may grow in response to loose stitches or towards the knot (Fig. 5.23). The area must be looked at carefully and steps taken to remove the suture and treat the inflammation.

The treatment of graft rejection must be prompt and in proportion to the threat, e.g. remove any loose sutures. If the signs are mild, increase, or re-start, topical steroids. Change from dilute to stronger preparations (guttae prednisolone, 1 per cent forte) and increase the frequency up to hourly. If the signs are moderate, increasing the strength and frequency should be accompanied by an orbital floor injection of steroid (usually as a soluble preparation such as betamethasone, 4 mg.). If the situation is acute and the rejection process well established, it is our practice to admit the patient and give them 500 mg methyl prednisolone intravenously, in addition to the above. If there are no problems following the infusion, the patient may be allowed home and reviewed frequently.

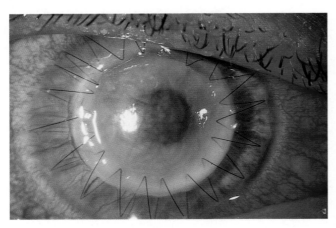

Figure 5.23. Intense neovascularization of the graft–host junction with deep vessels growing along the suture track and the interface.

Hourly steroid drops and nocturnal steroid ointment are maintained for about a week and reduced according to response. By the end of a month most patients will be using their medication four times a day. The reduction in intraocular inflammation may not, at least initially, be accompanied by any reduction in clarity of the graft. It seems that the endothelial cells need longer to recover from the effects of the smothering keratic precipitates. If the inflammation has been contained, clearing can be expected to occur over the next few weeks. In some eyes this never happens and the eye will need to be re-grafted.

In eyes which are particularly high risk, i.e. multiple previous grafts, perforation following infection, vascularized corneas and in those with serious ocular surface disease, tissue typing and systemic immunosuppression will need consideration.

GLAUCOMA

Glaucoma is of major prognostic significance for any grafted eye. It is well recognized that the chances of that graft failing are greatly increased if the pressure is not brought quickly under control. If there is no response to 'simple' topical medication, e.g. topical beta-blocker, control of pressure should be attempted with acetazolamide until surgery can be undertaken.

Glaucoma drainage is not a straightforward procedure in these eyes and usually either cytotoxic augmentation or tubal implantation is required. The development of a reliable diode laser should prove invaluable, avoiding surgery in eyes which have already suffered many interventions. The laser can be dosed and treatment repeated if there is insufficient response.

Pseudophakic bullous keratopathy will recur in any eye in which the causative lens has not been removed. If the visual return is known to be very poor, even if the cornea was completely clear, patient comfort will be the goal. Keratoplasty may do just that, but there is increasing evidence of the usefulness of amniotic membrane transplantation in improving the comfort and appearance of these eyes.

Section Three

Special Cases

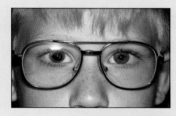
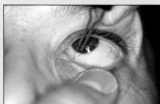

Chapter 6

The damaged paediatric eye

INTRODUCTION

The management of ocular trauma in children poses special problems above those faced by injuries in adults. Preoperative assessment of the child may be inadequate due to a poor and incomplete history and problems in examining an uncooperative patient. Any repair must be secure enough to withstand rubbing fingers and yet accurate to ensure rapid visual rehabilitation.

Trauma is the most common cause of unilateral blindness in the paediatric population. Blindness may be caused by the injury itself or by untreated strabismic or aphakic amblyopia. In major injuries, visual rehabilitation must be rapid and the danger of amblyopia is always present. There is a continued debate as to the role of intraocular lenses in the primary management of traumatic aphakia but attempts to correct aphakia with contact lenses are often associated with poor compliance, and so lens implantation offers many advantages.

Although the majority of accidental eye trauma will have been caused by other children, young boys left alone with dangerous toys and tools will often find ways of coming to harm on their own. Sporting injuries are also common; in the USA, baseball, ice hockey, street hockey and basketball are all well represented. Projectiles, such as darts, stones and glass, as well as sharp stabbing instruments such as pencils and scissors, are the most usual causes of damage (Fig. 6.1).

GENERAL MEASURES

History taking

A child who has suffered an eye injury may be frightened and in pain or shock. These feelings may be accentuated by the sights and sounds of an accident and emergency department. The child will be accompanied by a parent or adult who may be even more upset. Feelings of guilt

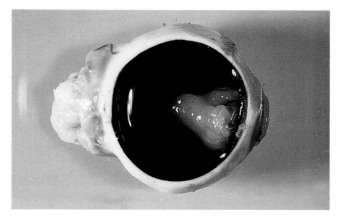

Figure 6.1. The result of giving a set of chisels to a seven-year-old boy for his birthday.

and blame are often close to the surface. A calm, softly-lit examination room, without a throng of observers, will encourage the child to settle. The presence of a nurse, experienced in counselling children, will help the consultation and offer a continuation of care after the initial examination.

It is crucial to take as full a history as possible, both from the child and any witness and carer/parent. Apart from detailing the injury itself, it is important to record any pre-existing ophthalmological problems and ascertain the patient's tetanus status. The final story of what actually happened may never be known. Sometimes, years later, the patient, now an adolescent or adult, may finally admit to what really occurred. The fear of retribution often creates a wall of silence.

Examination

As with all patients, it is important to establish visual acuities. In the child under two, this will involve fixation behaviour and preferential looking tests. In the older patient, picture or letter-matching will be more appropriate. Involving the parent in these assessments will often increase their reliability.

Examination of the child should begin with a careful search for other non-ophthalmic injuries. The eye and peri-orbita should be examined in a systematic fashion. Orbital blow-out fractures are not infrequent and may lead to trap-door inferior rectus entrapment in a quarter of cases. Fractures of the orbital roof are more common in children than in adults. Any orbital injury may be the cause of orbital cellulitis but in small children the infection may track intracranially, leading to a septic meningitis.

Small perforating eyelid lesions may appear innocuous. They may, however, be the entry wound of a retained intraocular, intraorbital or intracranial foreign body, or the track of a sharp perforating instrument that may have damaged the same structures (Figs 6.2a–d). A thorough examination to identify any posterior extension of the lid wound into the orbit is mandatory.

Plain X-rays or CT scanning must be used to exclude the possibility of intracranial foreign bodies. If this is a possibility the child should be covered prophylactically with antibiotics. Wood and most organic material is radiolucent, so there should be a lower threshold for exploring a wound if that is a risk.

Where there is lower canalicular damage, an orbital fracture with entrapment, or in cases of secondary infection, the child should be referred to an experienced sub-specialist. The management of complex lid and orbital trauma is beyond the scope of this book.

Examination of the eye itself may be difficult in the young child. The child may need to be examined under general anaesthesia (GA) to establish the exact nature of the injury.

Signs of globe rupture include loss of fullness and contour in the upper lid, an irregular or peaked pupil and a collapsed anterior chamber. A subconjunctival haemorrhage may mask a scleral rupture or puncture. It may be possible to grade the extent of the injury at the slit-lamp (Table 6.1), but a full examination of the wound will not be possible until the child is anaesthetized. It is imperative to delineate the full extent of any wound. This may require opening the conjunctiva and dissecting back across the sclera, sometimes disinserting the extra-ocular muscles to explore possible extended damage.

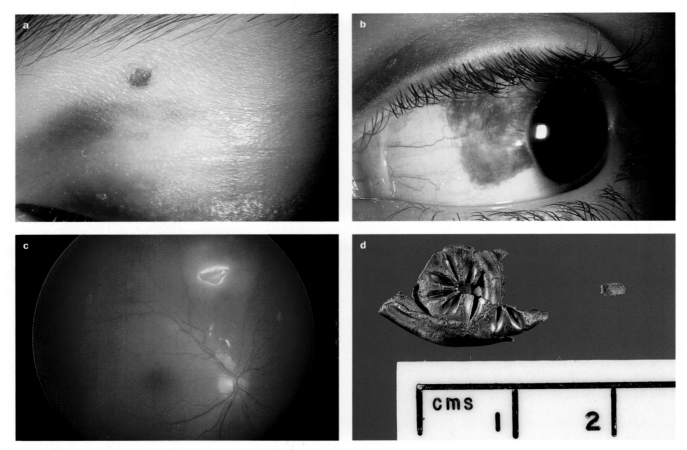

Figure 6.2. (a) Apparently innocuous wound, left upper eyelid. Note the marked bruising. (b) External eye picture showing conjunctival haemorrhage; the puncture mark of the sclera is covered by the upper lid. (c) Posterior segment photograph showing the tract taken by the foreign body with initial perforation and impact site. (d) The small fragment of cartridge casing that was removed from the retina.

Table 6.1. Grading ocular trauma in children.

Anterior, non-perforating	Conjunctival lacerations and haematomata
	Corneal abrasions
	Hyphaema
	Iridodialysis
	Ciliary body disinsertion
	Lens subluxation and traumatic cataract
Anterior, penetrating	Retained intraocular foreign body in the anterior or posterior segment
Anterior, perforating	The causative agent has entered the eye and then been withdrawn, e.g. a stick or nail, or where a foreign body has passed through the eye and now lies extraocularly.
Posterior segment	Mid-segment rupture
	Perforations either via the anterior segment or directly through the sclera
	Vitreous haemorrhage
	Retinal detachment/dialysis
	Retinal commotio (Berlin's oedema)
	Choroidal rupture

Non-accidental injury (NAI)

Any childhood injury can be non-accidental. Three to four per cent of children presenting to an ophthalmic emergency centre in the UK will have been mistreated. Forty per cent of abused children will have some form of ocular damage. Eighty per cent of children dying as a result of abuse will have ocular lesions. Abusing parents may have a characteristic psychological profile including a history of having been abused themselves, drug abuse, be of a young age (under 17), single and socially isolated. Whilst sometimes difficult in the face of a polished act, a thorough history from both parents independently can often establish inconsistencies which may alert the physician's suspicions.

Numerous ocular injuries have been reported to occur with non-accidental damage. These include peri-orbital haematomata, eyelid lacerations, subconjunctival haemorrhage, hyphaema and ciliary body disinsertion, traumatic lens subluxation and dislocation, iridodialysis, vitreous and pre-retinal haemorrhage, retinal dialysis and detachment, optic nerve atrophy and papilloedema.

A general examination may reveal bruising, bite-marks, cigarette burns and genital injuries. A petrified, withdrawn and highly anxious child should be a concern. A full skeletal survey looking for epiphyseal–diaphyseal distraction, rib or skull fractures and particularly multiple occult fractures at different stages of healing suggests a diagnosis of NAI. Intracranial haemorrhage is best diagnosed by magnetic resonance imaging.

Suspicions should be aroused if the history amongst witnesses and parents is inconsistent, if there are retinal haemorrhages, periocular bruising and lid lacerations or if there is an unexplained lens dislocation or cataract.

Unexplained conjunctival or corneal damage, especially that affecting the lower half of the eye, should also be of concern.

Team approach

The management of ocular trauma in children requires co-ordination between the surgeon, parents, nursing staff, optometrists, orthoptists, paediatricians and a dedicated paediatric anaesthetist.

Because the child may be too young to complain of specific problems, and as these problems may be subclinical to them, the child's follow-up must be carefully scheduled. For some this will simply involve regular orthoptic follow-up to monitor vision and for others this will require regular examinations under GA to check IOP or remove sutures.

Parents and carers play a pivotal role in the management of these children. If they have a firm understanding of why their child has had or is having a particular treatment, and they can appreciate the potential problems with non-compliance, your approach is more likely to succeed. Regular update sessions detailing the future visits and the progress that has been made will reinforce this 'partnership of care'.

Clinic visits should be as atraumatic as possible. Encouragement and reassurance are more readily accepted if they come from a member of staff the child knows. Continuity of care is even more important than with adults. Children as young as three or four will allow IOP checks in the clinic, using non-contact or applanation tonometry. The less painful and scary the consultation, the more co-operation will be had the next time.

Amblyopia

In children under seven, media opacities and anisometropia can lead to amblyopia. Ocular trauma may lead to both (see traumatic cataract management below). Unless special attention is directed towards treating or preventing amblyopia, the efforts of reconstructive surgery will be wasted with regard to vision. Patching regimens or the use of atropine penalization can be equally effective. Details of the possible protocols are beyond the scope of this book but a close liaison with optometric and orthoptic colleagues is recommended.

NON-PERFORATING INJURIES

Simple, minor injuries

Subconjunctival haemorrhage and superficial corneal abrasions are treated with reassurance and conservative medical treatment, respectively. Corneal foreign bodies may be removed at the slit-lamp in cooperative patients. Flecks of paint and dust may be simply wiped off the eye using a damp cotton bud.

Traumatic hyphaema

Hyphaema is a common complication of blunt ocular trauma in children. Damage to the iris root, stroma or sphincter can lead to anterior chamber haemorrhage. The extent and severity of the hyphaema will dictate the speed of its clearance from the anterior chamber. The potential risks from blood in the anterior chamber include secondary glaucoma, corneal staining and subsequent amblyopia. The causative blow can lead to varying degrees of ciliary body disinsertion, seen as angle recession in its milder forms due to the appearance on gonioscopy.

Hyphaema is treated with rest and dilute topical steroids. With large bleeds, or if the individual is particularly active and the instruction to rest at home is likely to be ignored, it is more sensible for the child to be treated in hospital. Rebleeding increases the risks of secondary complications.

Although raised IOP may complicate any hyphaema, it is more common with larger collections. The increased pressure may force blood pigments across the corneal endothelium into the stroma where it can stain the tissue a buff colour. It may take months or even years to clear.

Persistent elevation of IOP may compromise the optic nerve, although the degree and duration required to lead to a permanent damage is unknown.

Surgery should be avoided if at all possible. Medical treatment with topical beta-blockers and systemic acetazolamide are used in the first instance. With conservative management, over 95 per cent of cases will settle and have a visual acuity of 6/9 or better.

Where raised pressure complicates hyphaema in a child with sickle-cell disease, the surgeon should have a lower threshold for surgical intervention and undertake an anterior chamber washout. This should preferably be done within the first 48 hours if the hyphaema is not clearing significantly. These children often have large or complete ('8-ball') hyphaemas and their systemic disease contraindicates the use of carbonic anhydrase inhibitors. The risks of general anaesthesia in these children should be discussed in detail with the parents and medical colleagues. Tranexamic acid (given as a syrup at a dose of 25 mg/kg, 2–3 times a day) can reduce the risk of rebleeding.

Blunt trauma may cause ciliary body disinsertion. The classical teaching is that extensive angle involvement, affecting over half of the circumference, may lead to long-term problems with glaucoma. There is little evidence however, that this is a long-term problem in children. In children, the incidence of traumatic instability of the lens is less than that seen in adults where a third will also have zonular damage.

The surgical management of traumatic cataract is considered below.

PERFORATING INJURIES

Perforating injuries may be classified into simple, corneal injuries, mid-segment injuries and posterior segment perforation. The majority of children suffering simple, corneal perforation without lens involvement will have a final visual acuity of 6/9 or better. Mid-segment injuries, i.e. those between the corneo-scleral limbus and the pars plana (4–5 mm posterior to the limbus), usually result in vitreous loss. This complication can lead to secondary retinal traction and detachment (dialysis) and the liberation of pigment epithelial cells which can lead to proliferative vitreo-retinopathy. Traumatic cataract is also frequently seen in these eyes. Patients with mid-segment damage have a worse prognosis than those with simple anterior perforations.

A bandage contact lens will smooth the corneal surface making the eye feel more comfortable. This will allow a better and earlier post-operative examination and encourages visual rehabilitation.

If a cataract has developed, or is at risk of developing due to capsule perforation, lens surgery should be performed at the time of primary repair (see below). This is especially important in children under 7, who will be at risk of developing amblyopia. In children over 7, cataract surgery can be tackled as a secondary procedure.

Special considerations concerning primary repair in children

Anaesthesia for intraocular surgery in children requires extra care. The choroid fills a proportionately larger fraction of the posterior segment in children than in adults. Small fluctuations in heart rate, which will have a relatively greater effect on cardiac output, can dramatically affect the volume of the choroid. As the choroid swells with blood it will tend to displace the vitreous, which can make cataract surgery and wound closure more difficult. It is important for the child to be anaesthetized by an experienced paediatric anaesthetist with whom you have a close understanding. The level of anaesthesia should be maintained until surgery is completely finished.

The surgical techniques for children vary as much as they do for adults. You should try and preserve all viable tissue. Remove only ischaemic iris, conserving as much as possible. Excessive iris excision will result in photophobia and glare. Presenting vitreous should be excised with sponge and scissors to the level of the wound, to clear all anterior connections, thus avoiding traction.

Children have an exaggerated healing response and consequently care should be taken when positioning corneal sutures and how long they remain in the eye. Suture bites in the visual axis should be avoided; shorter central bites can be combined with longer peripheral bites to reduce central scarring and astigmatism (as discussed in Chapter 2). In children, the healing process may be florid.

Corneal sutures should be removed as early as possible, before the development of a vascularized scar which may lead to a permanent corneal opacity (Fig. 6.3).

Eccentric or para-axial corneal opacities from previous trauma can be managed by a rotational autograft (see Chapter 2). This technique works well in children and, because of the rapid healing response, sutures can be safely removed at three months. Primary corneal grafting may be necessary if the laceration is very large, crosses the visual axis or if the wound edges are macerated with evidence of tissue loss.

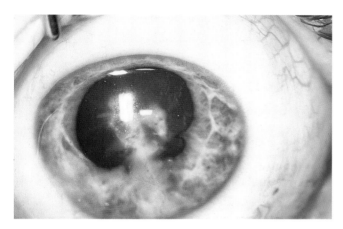

Figure 6.3. Vascularized corneal scar in the eye of a three-year-old girl who defaulted from follow-up. She re-presented with a densely amblyopic eye with loose, infected corneal sutures.

TRAUMATIC CATARACT

Some cataracts are partial and some may clear spontaneously. Opacities associated with capsular rupture are very unlikely to clear and often progress rapidly (Fig. 6.4). Cataracts can be diagnosed by the appearance of the red-reflex, although assessing the effect they may have on a child's vision is more difficult. Preferential-looking techniques can guide a surgeon as to the progression of any visual impairment but may be misleading when used as the sole determinant of whether surgery should be considered. Children with a best-corrected binocular acuity below 6/18 will find it difficult to function at school and surgery should be contemplated at an earlier stage.

The surgeon should have a lower threshold for surgery in the younger child, especially one under four years of age. Surgery will mark the first step in the long process of visual rehabilitation. Without a co-ordinated occlusion regimen, cataract removal can lead to more problems than not operating in the first place.

Management of aphakia in children

The options that are currently used to manage paediatric aphakia are aphakic glasses, contact lenses and IOLs. Epikeratophakia has been attempted in the past but problems with the availability of lenticules and post-operative healing have led to the abandonment of this procedure. Aphakic glasses are inexpensive and can be used at any age. They are easily changed to account for the refractive changes that follow surgery. They cannot be used for unilateral cataracts, however, as they will lead to intolerable differences in image size between the two eyes (aniseikonia). They also lead to reduced visual field and significant spherical and prismatic aberrations. The difficulties of seeing through aphakic glasses can lead to frustration in children (Fig. 6.5)

Contact lenses offer less magnification, fewer aberrations, greater visual field and better prospects for stereopsis. They cost more than aphakic glasses and have problems with compliance and hygiene. The majority of traumatic cataracts occur in boys from the age of three onwards. This coincides with the age above which contact lenses are poorly tolerated for unilateral aphakia.

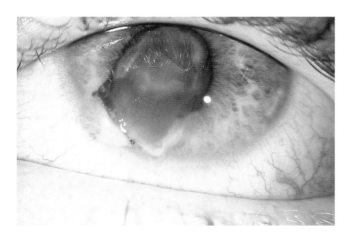

Figure 6.4. A six-year-old boy fell on a pair of scissors. The photograph shows prolapsed iris and a traumatic cataract.

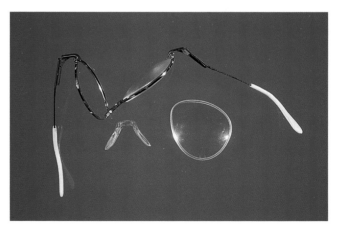

Figure 6.5. The result of a temper tantrum in a child with aphakic glasses.

Compliance with the wearing and hygiene of contact lenses is rarely excellent in the developed world. These problems are understandably magnified many times in the developing world where the cost of lost lenses has even more impact. IOL implantation offers the best option for the treatment of paediatric aphakia. The correction is full time and permanent. Previous concerns regarding the long-term stability of the biomaterial, refractive drift and post-operative inflammation have been allayed with recent advances.

Cataract surgery in children

The skills required for cataract removal and IOL implantation in children are those which are learned for adult surgery. Operations in children are, however, associated with particular problems in the pre-, per- and post-operative periods, especially in patients under two years of age (see Table 6.2).

WOUND CONSTRUCTION

Because children will tend to rub their eyes no matter how much they are told not to, a self-sealing scleral-tunnel wound, or a corneal wound with a long internal route, is preferred. The internal opening of the tunnel needs to be just wide enough to allow access for the aspiration device. The phaco-emulsifier is hardly ever needed, so the 2.8 mm keratome will make too big a hole. The choice of the IOL will determine the length of the final wound.

Because there is no nuclear rotation or fragment manipulation, a paracentesis could be perceived as redundant. In fact, a bimanual approach, with infusion and aspiration through two corneal stab incisions, is the technique of choice. The instruments can be swapped around to enable more complete removal of lens material.

During surgery, all incisions can become stretched such that they may leak. To be safe, a 10-0 absorbable suture can be used to close the incisions. A 10-0 nylon suture can be used but this will need removal after two weeks or so. A loose suture remaining in the eye of a child that is not brought back for regular checks can be a source of infection. Small incision surgery reduces the problems of high and fluctuating intravitreal pressure.

ANTERIOR CAPSULE

An anterior capsulotomy can be fashioned by manually tearing (CCC), nibbling with a vitrector (vitrectorrhexis) or cutting with endodiathermy (Fig. 6.6). The latter two techniques leave an irregular rim, which can increase the risk of capsular tears. In children, however, this risk is probably very small.

If an IOL is to be implanted, a circular capsulorrhexis is the anterior capsulotomy of choice. In traumatic cataract, there may be a hole in the anterior (and posterior) capsule which will not be visible until some lens matter has been aspirated (Fig. 6.7). Vision blue (Porc Ophthalmic Research, Netherlands) may help to define the edges of a tear.

Anterior capsular tears should be converted into smooth-edged arcs. Tearing a 'rhexis in a child's eye can be difficult. The use of high-density viscoelastics and a small incision will create sufficient anterior capsular pressure to prevent the tear working too peripherally. It is better to aim to tear a small 'rhexis as this will usually extend as it is torn. Folding over a flap and tearing as for an adult will result in losing the 'rhexis peripherally. If this is a threat, change the direction of pull on the anterior capsule flap towards the centre of the lens. This will rescue the tear.

Table 6.2. Particular problems with paediatric cataract surgery.

Pre-operative period
Late diagnosis
No biometry or keratometry
Systemic disorders including prematurity

Per-operative period
Small eye with a small pupil
Low scleral rigidity and high intra-vitreal pressure with marked fluctuation
Elastic anterior capsule
IOL power and physical size

Post-operative period
Uveitis
Posterior capsule opacification (PCO)
Induced myopia and other refractive changes
Glaucoma

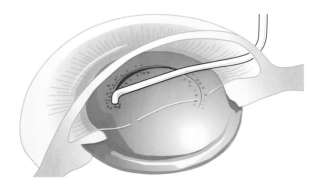

Figure 6.6. Drawing showing the use of the endodiathermy probe to cut the anterior capsule.

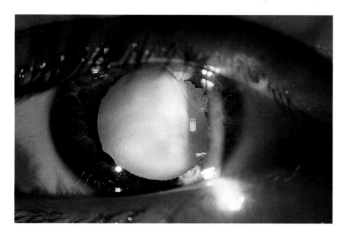

Figure 6.7. The anterior capsular details are invisible in this child's eye who has suffered a blunt injury.

An alternative technique is to make a linear, tangential incision in the anterior capsule between the top one-third and bottom two-thirds of the vertical diameter. The flap is grasped and pulled vertically downwards, towards 6 o'clock. Once the tear has 'crowned' the pull is brought in the diametrically opposite direction towards 12 o'clock. This will complete the tear (the so-called 'bucket-handle' technique – Figs 6.8a–e).

REMOVAL OF LENS MATERIAL

Hydrodissection is not required to allow the nucleus to be rotated and phaco-emulsified. It does, however, increase the efficiency of removal of the remaining lens material. This, in combination with crossing-over of infusion and aspiration instruments, allows a more complete clearance. This in turn may reduce the incidence of posterior capsular opacification (PCO).

POSTERIOR CAPSULE

Virtually 100 per cent of children having cataract extraction will go on to develop PCO. The resulting fibrosis may be florid, making manual, surgical capsulotomy difficult. Traction on the capsule at the time of this secondary surgery may lead to bleeding from the ciliary body. If thick, even a horizontally mounted Nd:YAG laser will have difficulty cutting a large enough hole.

It is undoubtedly better to prevent rather than treat PCO. Tearing a small anterior CCC, performing a careful lens material clear-out and placing an appropriate IOL (see below) into the capsular bag will all reduce PCO rates.

Despite these efforts, however, fibrosis can occur and many surgeons now routinely perform a primary posterior capsulorrhexis (PPCCC).

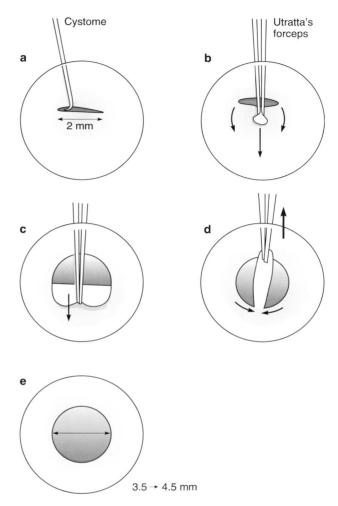

Figure 6.8. (a–e) Drawings showing the 'bucket-handle' technique for tearing a CCC in a child.

The posterior capsule (PC) is more fibrous and less elastic and thus behaves more like adult anterior capsule. To start a PPCCC, nick the capsule centrally with the cystotome. Injecting a small amount of viscoelastic through the gap makes the subsequent tearing easier. It also pushes the anterior vitreous face backwards. Once the PPCCC is complete, a very limited anterior vitrectomy will prevent the problems some authors have described with opacification of the anterior vitreous face. If PC tearing is difficult or if there is a puncture/rupture as a result of the initial trauma, the vitrector can be used. Alternatively, the endodiathermy probe can also be used.

Once both 'rhexes have been completed, the IOL can be implanted. Use heavy viscoelastic to keep the vitreous back out of the way of the leading haptic. Once the IOL is in the bag, gentle posterior pressure with a hook can herniate the optic through the PPCCC, thus capturing it centrally. This offers greater long-term IOL stability and can prevent posterior capsulophimosis (Figs 6.9a and b).

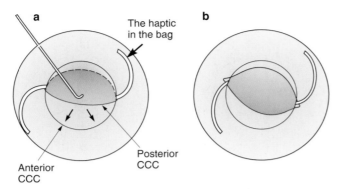

Figure 6.9. (a, b) Optic capture in a posterior capsulorrhexis (button-holing).

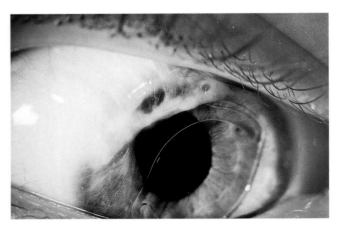

Figure 6.10. The eye of an eight-year-old boy who had cataract surgery with implantation. An oversized AC IOL was chosen to allow for growth in the child's eye. The tip of the proximal haptic can be seen lying subconjunctivally. The vision at presentation in 1989 was 6/6 and in January 2001 remained at this level. The lens is stable but continues to be a cause for concern.

INTRAOCULAR LENS IMPLANTATION

The two major problems which face a surgeon wanting to implant an IOL in a child are that the eye is physically small and will grow and that, with age, there will be a degree of myopic drift, which is more difficult to predict in very young children.

The average newborn baby has an eye that is 17 mm long and has a crystalline lens that is 6 mm in diameter. The comparable figures in an adult are 23–24 mm and 9.3 mm. Ninety per cent of the eye's growth will be complete by the time the child turns two years old. A vivid example of a misguided understanding of this growth is seen in Fig. 6.10.

Rigid all-PMMA lenses have been used since implantation in children's eyes began in the 1950s. Adult lenses have an optic of 6–7 mm diameter with a total size of 12–13 mm. Infants eyes are probably too small for these lenses but by the age of one they have probably grown sufficiently. There are reduced-size PMMA lenses available (5–6 mm optic and 10–12 mm total diameter) which can be used in very young children. Some surgeons advocate the use of heparin-surface modification (HSM – Pharmacia & Upjohn Ltd) to reduce post-operative inflammation.

Acrylic foldable lenses (particularly the Alcon Acysof IOL) are now being used extensively in surgery for paediatric cataract, whether as a result of trauma or a developmental abnormality. The vaulting, allowing increased optic/posterior capsule contact, and square-edge design of these lenses have led to a significant reduction in PCO rates in adults and children. The advantage of a foldable lens are that the incision can be kept smaller, which is safer in children and allows quicker visual rehabilitation.

The choice of dioptric power of the IOL causes difficulties. The surgeon can assume that the eye will grow and under-correct accordingly – 20 per cent off the power for children under two and 10 per cent for children between 2 and 8 years of age is one approach. Alternatively, the surgeon can implant the strength of lens indicated by on-the-table biometry and keratometry. This may be appropriate for the child at the time of operation but will be too strong as the eye grows. There will be an induced myopia that will need correction by spectacles, contact lens or secondary surgery, either lens exchange or 'piggy-backing'. The surgical advances in this secondary surgery may mean that this latter approach will become more common. If committed to regular lens exchange as the child grows, the lens style must be one that can easily be removed.

Post-operative management

Children can exhibit florid post-operative inflammation, hence subconjunctival and intensive topical steroids are advised. In some cases, where compliance is a potential problem, oral steroids can be used in the early post-operative period and if inflammation appears to increase. If dense fibrinous membranes form in the anterior chamber, some authors advocate the use of intracameral streptokinase.

If the injury has damaged the anterior capsule, the optic may work its way out of the bag and may lead to pupillary capture. This will often be associated with PCO. A posterior capsulotomy with anterior vitrectomy may be required.

If the child is too young to allow IOP checks in clinic, regular examinations under GA should be arranged. An early onset of glaucoma after surgery is usually caused by pupil block or peripheral anterior synechiae formation. Because of the risk of post-operative uveitis, it is probably best practice to perform a peripheral iridectomy in all children who have had complicated cataract surgery or where there is a breach in the remaining anterior capsule. Lifelong follow-up should be arranged.

REFRACTION

Traumatic cataracts are often unilateral and the optical balance between the phakic and pseudophakic eye can consequently be a challenge (see Chapter 5). Bifocal glasses are well tolerated by children with unilateral pseudophakia if there is no significant anisometropia. The upper border of the additional segment does not need to bisect the pupil as it does in an accommodative esotropia (Fig. 6.11). The full correction should be ordered and tried as this will form the basis for any occlusion treatment that may be required for amblyopia treatment or prevention.

A contact lens can be used as a short-term treatment for intolerable anisometropia but this approach will have all the problems of contact lens treatment for aphakia (see above). An intraocular lens exchange or addition will usually be required as a permanent solution.

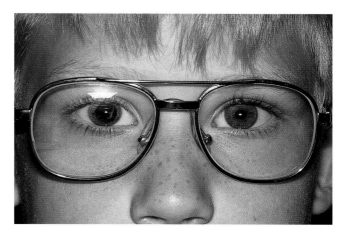

Figure 6.11. A six-year-old boy wearing bifocal glasses for unilateral pseudophakia following trauma.

Chapter 7

Ocular surface reconstruction

INTRODUCTION

This chapter will concentrate on the practical aspects of treatment. The surgical options for ocular surface reconstruction are still novel and some continue to be evaluated and developed.

The concept of the 'ocular surface' proposed by Thoft and Friend in 1977 (Table 7.1) has encouraged a fresh look at the biology and possible therapies for this important part of the eye. Internationally, damage to the ocular surface is a major cause of world blindness; xerophthalmia from vitamin A deficiency and trachoma remain potent problems in the developing world. In the developed world, chemical injuries, developmental abnormalities (e.g. aniridia) and immunological disease (e.g. cicatricial pemphigoid) cause most of the clinical disease.

The 'ocular surface' is made up of the epithelial surface of the eye covered by the tear film. This moist, slippery surface, which stretches from behind the grey line at the lid margin across the whole eye, is maintained in a healthy state by its supporting tissues, including glandular structures and sensory nerves. A stable tear film is vital to help maintain comfort and to help prevent infection. Together they work to maintain corneal clarity and health. All of these tissues are interdependent on each other and this microenvironment behaves as an ecosystem; damage to one structure will affect the health and function of other components.

Subjected to the constant trauma of blinking and rubbing, both conjunctival and corneal epithelia need rapid

renewal. The new cells are derived from stem cells. Stem cells are stable, pluripotential cells with a very low rate of division and few cellular markers. Their daughter cells however have the potential for rapid cellular division and, as they divide, the cells express characteristic markers indicating their maturation and differentiation. The anatomical arrangement of the two stem cell populations on the surface of the eye is quite different. Whereas the conjunctival stem cells are thought to be concentrated at the fornices, the corneal stem cells lie packed at the limbus, buried deep in the palisades of Vogt. These cells are densely grouped together and are concentrated at the superior and inferior limbus where the palisades are most clearly defined. This area of the corneal limbus is highly metabolically active, underlining the rapid rate of division of the daughter cells (transient amplifying cells). These cells differentiate into post-mitotic (wing) cells, and then move centribasally and centripetally to repair the corneal surface (Fig. 7.1).

In addition to being the seat of these cells, the limbus behaves as a barrier, inhibiting vascularization and migration of conjunctival epithelium onto the cornea. In disease, this barrier effect is lost, resulting in a characteristic clinical picture of an unstable, opaque corneal surface, with ingrowth of blood vessels (see Fig. 7.2 and Table 7.2).

Limbal stem cell deficiency

Limbal stem cell deficiency (LSCD) is the fundamental problem in ocular surface disease and many of the therapeutic aims are directed at correcting this.

The causes can be categorized into:

Type I: destruction or loss of the stem cells (Table 7.3).
Type II: loss or absence of the stromal supporting tissues or damage to the microenvironment, which supports the stem cells (Table 7.4).

Most conditions that cause ocular surface disease are bilateral and progressive, but may be asymmetric in severity; chemical injuries and other trauma may be unilateral.

Table 7.1. The ocular surface model of Thoft and Friend.

Components: conjunctival and corneal stratified, non-keratinized epithelia

Supporting structures – lids, tears, puncta

Dynamic interaction and interdependence occurs between all components

Limbus is a barrier between conjunctiva and corneal epithelia

Limbal stem cells have fundamental role

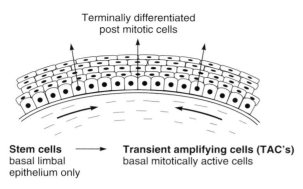

Figure 7.1. A diagram to show the normal maturation sequence and migration of corneal limbal stem cells. The arrows indicate centribasal and centripetal spread.

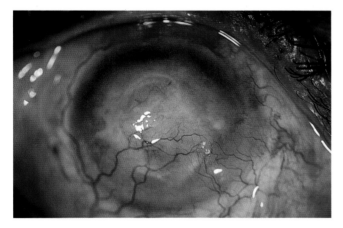

Figure 7.2. Characteristic appearance of an eye with severe stem cell deficiency. Note the vascularization, abnormal conjunctivalization of the cornea, persistent epithelial defect and chronic inflammation.

Table 7.2. The clinical signs of limbal stem cell deficiency.

Signs are caused by damage/death of limbal stem cells
Typical clinical signs include:
 Fibrovascular ingrowth
 Chronic inflammation
 Recurrrent epithelial defects
 Conjunctival epithelial ingrowth
 (Impression cytology confirms these changes)

Table 7.3. Limbal stem cell deficiency (LSCD) Type I – examples of conditions that cause destruction or loss of stem cells.

Chemical or thermal injuries
Stevens–Johnson syndrome
Multiple ocular surgery causing limbal damage, e.g. repeat retinal detachment or glaucoma operations.
Contact lens related, hypoxia or related to cleaning solutions
Sunshine/ultra-violet light
Microbial infection, severe and chronic

Table 7.4. Limbal stem cell deficiency (LSCD) Type II – examples of conditions associated with destruction of, or damage to, the supporting stroma/microenvironment of limbal stem cells.

Aniridia
Multiple endocrine deficiency
Chronic inflammation/ulceration
Peripheral keratitis
Neurotrophic keratitis
Pterygium/pseudopterygium

Table 7.5. Causes of conjunctival scarring.

Infective conditions: *Chlamydia trachomatis, Streptococcus pneumoniae*, diphtheroids, *Varicella* virus, acne rosacea
Autoimmune disease: ocular pemphigoid, Sjögren's syndrome, Stevens–Johnson syndrome.
Atopic disease
Chemical and thermal injuries
Multiple surgery
Topical ocular medications and preservatives:
– with benzylkonium, guanethidine, adrenaline (Ganda or dipiverfin).
(*Note*: the concentration of benzylalkonium chloride in Xalatan is 0.02 per cent, twice as high as in other medications).
– with thiomersal, contact lens solutions.

Conjunctival and lid disease

This can be caused by a variety of mediators shown in Table 7.5. Severe inflammation and chronic exposure to toxic chemicals causes permanent damage and scarring to the conjunctiva and its accessory structures. This may lead to scarring, loss of goblet cells, lacrimal glands and conjunctival stem cells. Scarring causes cicatricial entropion, secondary trichiasis, and symblepharon. A poor tear film combined with reduction of lysozyme levels further reduces the defences, and suppurative disease threatens whenever the corneal epithelium is damaged.

The importance of normal lid function and morphology must be stressed. The lids have to move normally in reflex blinking and close when sleeping. Paralysis associated with corneal anaesthesia is doubly compromising.

Cicatricial entropion (Fig. 7.3) or ectropion (Fig. 7.4) both produce poor corneal cover.

This new understanding of the ocular surface allows a clearer, strategic approach to therapy. By implication, therapy must be holistic and acknowledge this dynamic biological system. Thus surgical treatment can only be part of

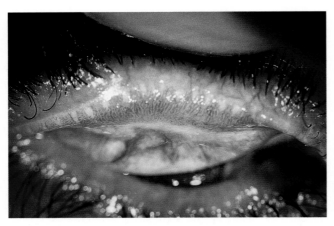

Figure 7.3. A case of trachoma showing an everted lid with marked cicatricial entropion.

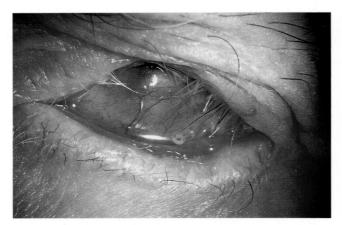

Figure 7.4. Ocular cicatricial pemphigoid producing both cicatricial entropion of the upper lid with trichiasis and lower lid ectropion.

any solution, and if an operation is to have a chance of success, it has to be undertaken respecting the other components of this 'ecosystem'; to ignore this principle is to invite failure. The approaches to treatment are still relatively crude but are beginning to achieve success in conditions not previously thought treatable. Further refinements are awaited.

HISTORY

Patients with established ocular surface disorders have usually had uncomfortable eyes for many years with symptoms of moderate to severe visual loss. They will often have sought many previous opinions in an attempt to find suitable treatment. Acute deterioration in their condition can occur due to mechanical trauma from ingrowing lashes, the development of a persistent corneal epithelial defect or infection, perhaps causing corneal perforation.

These patients are miserable and their lives become dominated by their eye symptoms and limitations.

The cause of the problem will be obvious when there is a history of assault or injury. In some, associated general or ocular disease will give a clue as to the aetiology, while in others greater deliberation will be required. A history of prolonged ocular medication should alert the ophthalmologist to the possibility that chronic exposure to the preservatives and active components could be the cause of the problem.

If there are any criminal or occupational issues to be considered, the history must include the exact timing of events and the involvement of any third party, as well as a record of the nature of the chemical or accident. This information is essential in both the immediate, post-injury phase and also later if the matter takes a legal course. Photographic documentation is most advisable for a complete accurate record.

You should record past and current treatments. This is important not only to determine which medications have already been tried and have failed but also because certain medications, be they topical or oral, can be the cause of the disease (Table 7.6).

DIAGNOSIS (see also Table 7.6)

Ocular surface disorders vary from mild to very severe. In the mildest forms the signs are subtle and therapy is usually straightforward, perhaps requiring nothing more than a change in medication. In the severe forms the findings are usually gross and the multiple problems will need a campaign of complex surgical and medical therapy.

The characteristic signs must be carefully sought with a mind to planning treatment, grading the findings in both eyes. Look systematically at the various components of the

Table 7.6. History – points to be considered.

Duration, recent or lifelong (e.g. congenital problems such as aniridia) Acute or chronic?

Ocular only? Enquire about possible systemic involvement

Systemic too? Ask for history of joint, mouth, skin, perineal problems, e.g. in pemphigoid

Occupational history: chemical and dust exposure

Injury: accidental/criminal; acid/alkali; contact lenses

Contact lenses: cleansing regimens, wearing times (hypoxia)

Family history: aniridia, atopy

Ocular medication: guanethidine, adrenaline, Ganda, dipiverfin, self-medications, e.g. 'eyebright'

Ocular preservatives: thiomersol, benzylkonium chloride

Systemic medications: practolol, sulpha drugs (Stevens–Johnson syndrome)

Therapies already tried: tear replacements, etc.

Past medical history: allergies/atopy

ocular surface and judge which are involved in the process; lids, tears, conjunctiva, limbus and cornea.

(1) Lids

Look for scarring, ectropion, entropion, pattern of blinking and closure and trichiasis.

(2) Tear film

Assess the tear film and corneal sensation before instilling any drops. A superficial punctate staining pattern occurs in dry areas of the cornea. Clinical tests such as Schirmer's strip testing and assessment of tear osmolarity can confirm tear film deficiencies. The tear film may be quantitatively assessed by doing a fluorescein clearance test (FCT) (see Table 7.7).

(3) Conjunctiva

Record all conjunctival scarring and the position of any symblepharon. Look particularly at the plica semilunaris; it is lost at an early stage in cicatricial conjunctival disease such as ocular pemphigoid.

(4) Cornea and limbus

Loss of the brilliance of the corneal reflex is quickly noted. Loss of the limbal barrier is characterized by the ingrowth of a fibrovascular pannus. This may be limited to a small zone of a few clock hours (a local breach in the 'defences') or total loss of integrity with 360 degree vascular ingrowth. A combination of loss of the limbal barrier and corneal epithelial problems spells major ocular surface difficulties. If corneal sensation is also diminished, neurotrophic keratitis results because of loss of neurotrophic growth factors, essential to corneal health.

Corneal disease can be divided into:
i) Mild: epithelial disturbances, blizzard keratopathy, punctate epithelial erosions (Fig. 7.5).
ii) Moderate: persistent epithelial defects, local loss of the limbal barrier effect (Fig. 7.6).

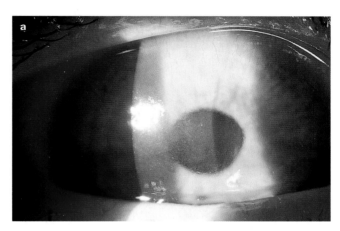

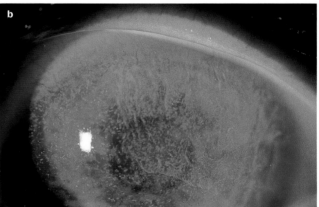

Figure 7.5. (a) Blizzard keratopathy in a patient with contact lens problem. (b) Same eye after instillation of fluorescein.

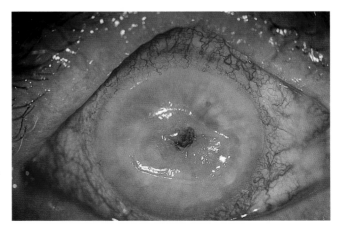

Figure 7.6. Moderate corneal disease in a case of ocular surface disease (OSD) showing a persistent epithelial defect.

Table 7.7. Technique of fluorescein clearance test (FCT).

To evaluate reflex tearing and tear clearance:

(1) Apply a drop of proxymethacaine and dry the conjunctival sac of each eye.

(2) Apply 5 microlitres of 0.25% fluorescein (one drop from a minims approximates this amount) and allow normal blinking

(3) Perform a Schirmer's test for 1 min at 10 and 20 min.

(4) At the end of 30 min, do a nasal stimulation test whilst the last Schirmer's test is done.

How to interpret a FCT
Basal secretion: normal if wetting length of first two strips > 3 mm.
Reflex secretion: normal if wetting length of last strip >first two strips.
Clearance: normal if the eye clears after the first strip.

iii) Severe: persistent epithelial defects, vascular pannus, scarring, usually in association with limbal disease, poor tear film and conjunctival scarring (Fig. 7.7).

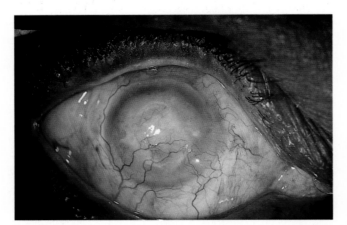

Figure 7.7. A case of severe corneal problems in a patient with OSD – note the vascular pannus due to loss of the limbal barrier effect.

(5) Intraocular pressure

Must be measured, remembering that secondary glaucoma is a poor prognostic indicator in ocular surface reconstruction.

(6) General condition

If systemic immunosuppression is to be used following reconstruction, enrol the help of a physician experienced in the supervision of such patients. These drugs are potentially dangerous and shared care gives both the ophthalmologist and the patient appropriate support.

The principles of the examination routine are summarized in Table 7.8.

Table 7.8. Examination routine for the ocular surface.

Lids: position, entropion, closure, blink pattern

Tears: production, conjunctivochalaisis, tear break-up time, mucous

Conjunctiva: symblepharon, active ulceration, keratinization, inflammation

Limbus: infiltration, vascularization, loss of 'barrier' (and extent of loss), ischaemia

Cornea: sensation, vascularization, mucous filaments, infection, scarring, perforation

Corneal epithelium: blizzard keratopathy, other epitheliopathy, e.g. punctate epithelial, poor wetting, instability, persistent epithelial defect.

Fellow eye: signs of involvement may be less marked. Can tissue be used from the fellow eye?

Other structures: iris, e.g. aniridia, previous buphthalmos, previous surgery to eye, other mucous membranes.

STRATEGIES FOR THE TREATMENT OF OCULAR SURFACE DISEASE

Attention must first be directed at controlling or correcting any underlying condition if this is possible. Surgical objectives can then be applied to replace stem cells, treat scar tissue, improve the local environment, and carry out corneal grafting and cataract surgery (see Tables 7.9 and 7.10).

Table 7.9. Strategies in ocular surface reconstruction.

(1) Treat underlying pathology: remove toxic causes, control infection and inflammation

(2) Restore or augment ocular defence mechanisms: tears, lids, lashes, conjunctival surgery

(3) Prevent or treat mechanical problems

(4) Modify limbal stromal environment: amniotic membrane transplantation, autologous serum eye drops

(5) Replace stem cells: limbal autografts (well established) or allografts (immunosuppression needed for survival of 75% @ two years, 50% @ five years)

(6) Combinations of all the above

(7) Additional surgery: including penetrating and lamellar keratoplasty, cataract surgery, keratoprosthesis.

Table 7.10. Surgical strategies for the treatment of ocular surface disease.

Ocular surface reconstruction (OSR): mild group
Remove only damaged limbus + peritomy

< 2 hours, use patch amniotic membrane transplant

> 2 hours, peritomy + AMT to cover defect

— use perilimbal rim of amniotic membrane (AM)

— suture to edge of corneal defect

OSR: moderate group
If uninflamed, strip ocular surface of pannus.

If inflamed, initial AMT cover (total or perilimbal)

Wait and see before deciding on limbal autografting (LAU)/limbal allografting (LAL)

LAL done as required

OSR: severe group
These eyes usually have multiple coexisting pathology

Surgery is usually staged and often multiple

Strip and remove vascular pannus

AMT + LAL + penetrating keratoplasty (PKP) + other surgeries such as cataract

Immunosuppress if combining LAL + PKP

Repeat/treat problems as they arise, e.g. AMT + further LAL + PKP, etc.

Use additional, supportive measures, including autologous serum eye drops, silicone bandage contact lenses

Treatment of the underlying condition

EXTERNAL IRRITANTS

Suspected medications should be discontinued, noting any improvement (see Figs 7.8a and b). The use of preservative-free drops is recommended wherever available.

INFECTIVE CAUSES

Aim to improve the local environment by treating infection with appropriate topical or systemic antibiotics. Acne rosacea should be treated aggressively in these cases; treatment involves a lid hygiene programme in conjunction with a six-week (minimum) course of tetracycline (e.g. doxycycline, 100 mg daily), or erythromycin, 250 mg three times daily.

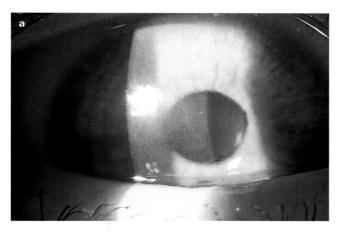

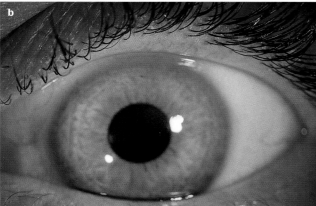

Figure 7.8. (a, b) The same case as in Fig. 7.5 of blizzard keratopathy showing spontaneous improvement of physical signs after avoiding lens wear and solutions.

Trachoma is now treated with a single dose of azithromycin (1 g in adults or 20 mg per kg for children). Sufficient coverage of the at-risk population is necessary to overcome the residual reservoir of infection within the community. Compliance and the opportunity to monitor treatment are much greater with azithromycin than previous treatment. This comprised oral tetracycline (in adults) or erythromycin (in children) both at 250 mg, four times a day in conjunction with topical treatment (tetracycline or oxytetracycline ointment).

AUTOIMMUNE CAUSES

Oculo-cutaneous diseases such as ocular cicatricial pemphigoid are intractable problems. Disease activity may be (partially) controlled by aggressive immunosuppression, given as early as possible in the process.

In ocular cicatricial pemphigoid, maintenance therapy with dapsone is useful, particularly when a conjunctival biopsy has demonstrated basement membrane linear IgA deposits. Ocular surface reconstruction should only be considered in desperate cases, as the surgical outcomes are poor even when the underlying condition is rendered quiescent with immunosuppression. In persistent cases, oral steroids, cyclosporin, cyclophosphamide (1–3 mg/kg per day) and azathioprine (1–3 mg/kg per day) may also be tried. In those cases resistant to oral treatment, pulses of methylprednisolone alone or with cyclosphosphamide and Mesna can be given at suitable intervals. The co-administration of Mesna (sodium 2-mercapto-ethanesulphonate) reduces the urotoxic effects of alkylating agents like cyclophosphamide. The baseline tests required and the treatment protocol are described in Tables 7.11a and b. The usefulness of topical cyclosporin has not been proven.

Table 7.11a. Routine checks before using pulsed cyclophosphamide with Mesna and methylprednisolone.

Exclude the presence of an infective element.

Baseline tests:

- Pulse, blood pressure, urinalysis (if blood or protein in urine, send mid-stream urine for microscopy to rule out a urinary tract infection).
- Full blood count (FBC) looking for myelosuppression, urea, electrolytes (U & Es) and creatinine (looking for urotoxic effects). Always wait for results before starting cyclophosphamide. If abnormal a physician needs to be consulted to decide if safe to proceed.
- Intravenous (IV) access is required with a Venflon (butterfly needle is inadequate in case of extravasation).
- Commence an IV drip of 1 litre of normal saline over 4 to 6 hours (can be infused at the same time as pulsed therapy). Encourage the patient to drink clear fluids (up to 2 litres) during the process. A good fluid intake and output reduces the risk of haemorrhagic cystitis from the cyclophosphamide.

Table 7.11b. Protocol for using pulsed cyclophosphamide with Mesna and methylprednisolone.

Time

0 hours:	Start the IV 500 mg methylprednisolone in a 250 ml bag of normal saline. Infuse over 2 hours. Give 400 mg of Mesna orally (1st dose is 2 hours prior to the cyclophospahmide infusion).
2 hours:	Give metoclopramide 10 mg IV (or ganesetron if problems with nausea). Start the IV cyclophosphamide at 10 mg/kg (in a 250 ml bag of normal saline, infusing over 2 hours).
6 hours:	Give another 400 mg tablet of Mesna (2nd dose is 2 hours post cyclophosphamide).
10 hours:	A 3rd dose of 400 mg Mesna is given orally (3rd dose is 6 hours post cyclophosphamide).

Patients take home:

● Oral anti-emetic, e.g. 10 mg metoclopramide 8 hourly as required (if problems with nausea).
● Amphotericin lozenges to take four times a day for 2 weeks (prophylaxis against candida).
● Ranitidine 150 mg twice daily (helps prevent dyspepsia from the steroid).
● Blood forms for testing FBC, U & Es and creatinine at 10 days post treatment.

Frequency:

● A total of up to six pulses is given. The first three pulses are given every two weeks.
● If disease not suitably controlled, then repeat the pulses at 2-weekly intervals.
● If improving, then the interval can be extended to monthly.

Restoring the ocular defence mechanisms

TEARS

Where they are insufficient, the options for treatment are (a) tear replacement or (b) tear conservation by punctal occlusion. Both approaches may be required or (c) other supportive therapies.

Tear replacement

Artificial lubricants come as drops, gels or slow-release inserts. It is important to use preservative-free preparations whenever possible. Topical sodium hyaluronate and topical cyclosporin are available and the latter is useful in the more refractory cases. Autologous serum seems to offer particular benefits, but because of problems in handling blood products their availability is not universal. When mucous strings, filamentary keratitis or plaque formation are seen, 5 or 10 per cent acetylcysteine drops (used five times a day) will break up the deposits and give symptomatic relief and resolution of clinical signs.

Tear conservation

Where production is reduced, and measured as such, punctal occlusion with cautery will achieve a lasting effect (Figs 7.9a and b). Silicone plugs and gelatin rods have their place when the diagnosis is unclear or if the patient is anxious, but their effects are often temporary.

In the first instance the puncta are closed with gelatin rods or silicone plugs. If the patient achieves significant improvement in their symptoms, then in these severe cases, permanent punctal occlusion is offered. The lower

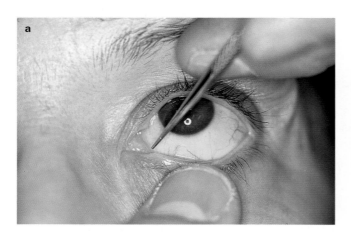 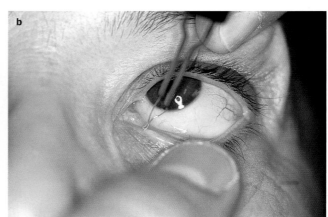

Figure 7.9. (a, b) Permanent punctal occlusion – dilatation of the lower punctum, followed by cautery to cause punctal closure.

are closed first, and depending on the response, the upper puncta can be closed at a later stage. Return of symptoms usually indicates that one or more of them have reopened; the process may then be repeated.

Supportive therapies

Include the use of autologous serum eye drops (containing chemical mediators capable of supporting stem cell and epithelial function), and immunosuppressive drugs such as cyclosporin A which help suppress underlying immunological processes and prevent rejection of any allografts. Some beneficial responses to topical cyclosporin A have been reported.

Autologous serum eye drops are simply prepared as follows:

(1) Draw 10–20 ml of blood into a plain (group and save) bottle.
(2) Centrifuge the blood at 1500 rpm for 5 min to form serum in the supernatant.
(3) Aliquot the serum into sterile 1 ml tubes.
(4) Dilute each tube with balanced salt solution to a final volume of 5 ml.
(5) Refrigerate this 20 per cent concentration solution in an eyedropper at 4–8°C, for the patient to use.
(6) Freeze the rest of the serum at −20°C until the next dilution.

Prevent or treat mechanical problems

Entropion, with or without lash problems, (trichiasis/distichiasis/metaplastic) causes the most severe problems. Ectropion tends to be less problematic and may not require any active treatment.

Treatment of entropion with lash problems:

(1) Epilation.
(2) Large bandage contact lens, to protect the corneal surface.
(3) Lubricants.

SURGICAL

Cryotherapy is usually helpful for in-turning lashes. Mild to moderate cicatricial entropion of the upper lid, with or without trichiasis, needs anterior lamella (skin and orbicularis) repositioning or a tarsal fracture procedure for the lower lids. In more severe disease, terminal tarsus rotation (e.g. Trabut-type procedure) may be required (see Figs 7.10a–d).

Where the posterior lamella (conjunctiva and tarsal plate) of the eyelid is shortened, a mucous membrane graft should be used when correcting the entropion. Levator recession will lower the lid, providing better corneal cover.

Where the disease is bilateral, an alternative source of mucous membrane must be used, and buccal or lip mucosa is satisfactory. The thicker, hard palate mucosa can be used on the tarsal conjunctiva and may be more resistant to recurrence. Alternatively mucous membrane may be harvested from the nasal turbinate. This mucous membrane has very similar histology to conjunctiva with plentiful goblet cells. The mucosa is sewn into the fornix.

More recently, reports of good results using amniotic membrane have been published.

Lagophthalmos: The problem of exposure must be clearly addressed. Lid taping is rarely sufficient and a tarsorrhaphy, either lateral or central, may be needed to achieve adequate corneal cover. Botulinum toxin injected into the levator palpebrae superioris (see Table 7.12) will cause a reversible ptosis, and allows easy examination of the cornea. Further surgical techniques needed to correct lid problems are best found in an oculoplastics manual.

Table 7.12. Technique of botulinum toxin-induced ptosis.

(1) Using an insulin syringe, load 20 units of botulinum toxin (e.g. 0.1 ml of Dysport).

(2) Inject into the centre part of the upper lid at the skin crease aiming to the roof of the orbit.

(3) The lid starts to drop at 1 to 3 days with maximum ptosis achieved at 3 to 12 days.

(4) Repeat injections may be required for full ptosis.

(5) The effect lasts an average of 12 weeks.

Side effects can be common, particularly diplopia due to superior and/ or lateral rectus weakness, but these tend to resolve completely.

SURGICAL APPROACHES

Amniotic membrane transplantation (AMT)

Amniotic membrane (AM) consists of a thick basement membrane (which encourages migration of epithelial cells and strong adhesion to the underlying corneal stroma) and an avascular, stromal matrix rich in growth and anti-apoptotic factors. This combination has the ability to improve the microenvironment of the cornea and limbus. By encouraging stem cell proliferation and reducing inflammation, re-epithelialization is enhanced.

AMT is now accepted as a valuable, additional arm of therapy. By using it as a preliminary step in ocular surface reconstruction (OSR), limbal stem transplantation may be avoided. Its wider applications include treating partial limbal stem cell loss: as a first stage in a series of procedures in OSR it has a positive influence on the survival and thus

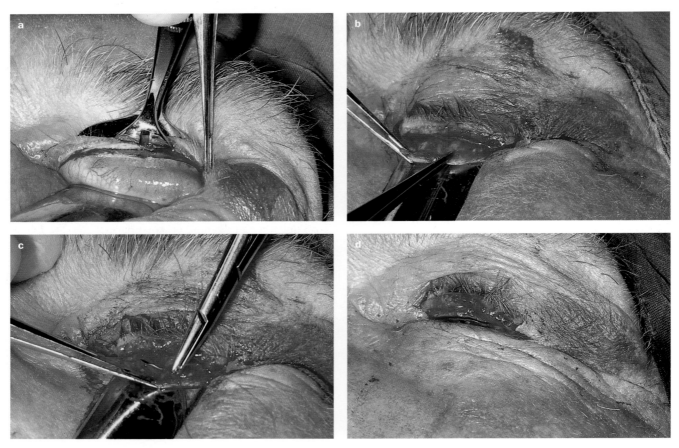

Figure 7.10. (a) Trabut-type procedure – the upper lid is everted with a lid clamp. (b) After rotation of the terminal tarsus, the posterior lamella is freed and advanced by recessing the levator muscle. (c) Three double-ended 4-0 catgut sutures are used to suture the anterior lamella (skin and muscle) to the anterior surface of the tarsus. Further sutures can be passed above, going through the conjunctiva and skin, at the upper border of the tarsal plate and the level of the skin crease. (d) At the end of the operation, the everted, lash-bearing skin is shown rotated clear of the new lid margin.

success of any second-stage procedures like stem cell grafting or penetrating keratoplasty; as a patch graft or as a bandage lens in cases of persistent epithelial defect (see Tables 7.13, 7.14 and 7.15). The steps of management of persistent epithelial defects (PEDs) are summarized in Table 7.16. AMT has also been used in conjunctival reconstruction, symptomatic bullous keratopathy, recurrent corneal erosions and as scleral patch grafts.

TECHNIQUE OF AMNIOTIC MEMBRANE TRANSPLANTATION

AMT is a straightforward procedure, the key to which is ensuring that the membrane is sutured stretched, so it drapes tightly. Whether it really matters which side should be used up or down is not clear, but it has been suggested that if the amniotic membrane is needed as a 'substrate' to support limbal cells, then it should be used *basement*

Table 7.13. Therapeutic properties of amniotic membrane.

Migration of epithelial cells facilitated by the thick basement membrane.

Adhesion of basal epithelial cells reinforced; cell density doubles.

Anti-apoptotic effect encourages epithelial survival.

Enhances transforming growth factor (TGFβ) production.

Promotes epithelial differentiation.

Reduces inflammation in the supporting tissues by absorbing cytokines.

Fibrovascular activity is inhibited.

Short/intermediate term effect only.

membrane side up; when needed as a biological bandage lens, it should be used *basement membrane side down.*

The amniotic membrane can be used as a patch graft for peripheral PEDs (Figs 7.11a and b), to provide central corneal cover (Figs 7.12a–c) or to provide total cover for the cornea and limbus (Figs 7.13a–d).

Table 7.14. Amniotic membrane transplantation (AMT) – beneficial effects in ocular surface reconstruction.

Encourages conjunctival cell cover of corneal surface; smooth, wettable, stable.

Produces marked reduction in inflammation of limbal tissues.

Reduces rate of rejection of limbal stem cell allografts, i.e.

< 14 per cent after AMT

> 75 per cent without AMT

Reduces need for immunosuppression

Table 7.15. Amniotic membrane transplantation – indications for use.

First stage of ocular surface reconstruction prior to stem cell allografting.

Acute chemical injury/burn.

To encourage epithelial cover of persistent epithelial erosions (patch graft).

Conjunctival defects, acute burns, symblepharon.

Surgical treatment of conjunctival cicatricial disease, total corneal + perilimbal cover.

Reduces discomfort in patients with bullous keratopathy (total corneal cover).

Pterygium surgery.

Table 7.16. Managing persistent epithelial defects.

Remove the source of mechanical trauma (e.g. trichiasis).

Discontinue steroids and benzyalkonium-preserved drops. Avoid aminoglycosides.

Establish level of tear production.

Use lubricants including sodium hyaluronate.

Bandage contact lenses.

Amniotic membrane transplantation.

Stem cell transplantation.

Tarsorrhaphy.

Conjunctival flap.

Give vitamin C, topical (10 per cent drops) and oral (1000 mg per day).

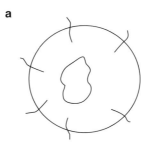
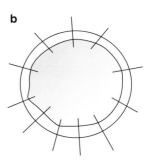
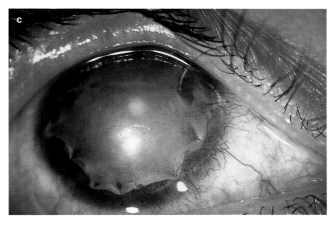

Figure 7.12. (a, b) Central corneal cover with an amniotic membrane. (c) A case of aniridia following amniotic membrane transplant for a persistent epithelial defect.

In the UK the membrane can be obtained from the North London Tissue Bank. It comes mounted on a 2 × 2 cm or 3 × 3 cm square of card and arrives 'basement membrane up' Confirm this by using a Weckcell sponge. The stromal side is stickier than the basement membrane side.

Procedure

The size of the AMT will depend on the pathology being treated. The material is easy to use and suture, and can be trimmed to size.

(1) Either local or general anaesthesia can be used.

(2) Perform a superficial keratectomy to denude the abnormal epithelium or fibrovascular pannus. Avoid sharp dissection if possible.

(3) If the whole cornea needs to be covered, a conjunctival peritomy plus recession to about 5 mm is done. A drop of phenylephrine, 10 per cent, can help reduce bleeding.

(4) Remove the membrane from the card and drape one end over the cornea.

(5) Begin suturing one side to anchor the membrane, using 10-0 vicryl or 10-0 nylon sutures.

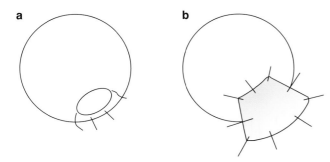

Figure 7.11. (a, b) Amniotic membrane used to patch a persistent epithelial defect (PED).

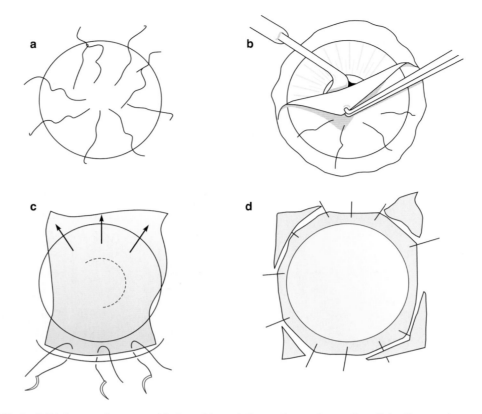

Figure 7.13. (a–d) Total cover of cornea and limbus with amniotic membrane after peeling off the fibrovascular pannus.

(6) Trim the membrane to approximately the required size and pull the AM taught as the opposite side is sutured in place. Continue suturing around the perimeter of the graft, keeping the AM taut. Trim off excess AM at the end.

(7) Make sure the suture ends are buried and cover with an appropriately sized bandage contact lens at the end of the procedure.

(8) Guttae maxitrol is given three times daily for four weeks, by which time the amniotic membrane is beginning to absorb.

Useful hints

(1) Create a partial-thickness groove in the cornea where it is thought that the outer limit of the membrane should be, using a trephine or diamond blade. This will give you anchor points for placing your sutures.

(2) Undersize the membrane slightly, as this will help stretch the membrane tight when suturing (loose AMTs tend to fall off).

(3) When suturing, use as long a bite as possible. This makes it easier to rotate and bury the knots and will make the eye more comfortable post-operatively.

Prevent loosening but you do need to rotate them even if a bandage lens is used.

Worked Example 7.1: A case of severe chemical injury treated with tenoplasty and amniotic membrane transplantation.

Case

A 9-year-old male received lime into his right eye whilst out playing with his friends. In A&E the eye was irrigated until the pH was neutralized. He was referred to the corneal service with severe limbal ischaemia and total corneal and inferior conjunctival epithelial loss – a Hughes grade III/IV chemical burn (Fig. 7.14 and 7.15).

Treatment: with vitamin C, doxycycline p.o., ascorbate and chloramphenicol drops. The clinical status deteriorated over five days and corneal melting threatened. Having discussed the options with his parents and the patient, he was taken to theatre.

Clinical findings

Only a superior 1.5 mm fringe of corneal epithelium, between 10 and 2 o'clock remained; conjunctival sloughing and signs of early corneal melting were present.

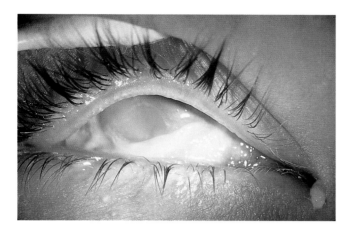

Figure 7.14. Anterior segment photo showing a cloudy cornea with limbal and conjunctival ischaemia following the alkali burn.

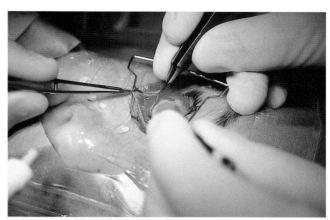

Figure 7.16. Tenon's capsule is identified and advanced to the limbus.

The conjunctival and corneal defect were covered with amniotic membrane (Fig. 7.17). The AM was brought up tight to the edge of the corneal epithelial fringe superiorly and sutured using 10-0 vicryl and a bandage contact lens was inserted.

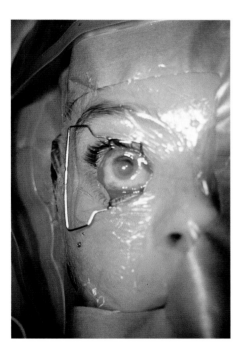

Figure 7.15. Note that three-quarters of the limbus is blanched and ischaemic.

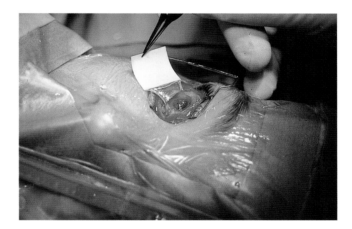

Figure 7.17. Amniotic membrane is peeled off its carrier card and sutured in place.

Procedure

The underside of the upper eyelid was inspected and scrubbed to remove any remaining particulate matter. The dead tissue around the edge of the cornea and the opaque corneal eithelium were debrided. A fresh edge of conjunctiva was defined and the Tenon's capsule was advanced up to the inferior limbus (tenoplasty) and sutured in place with 10-0 vicryl (Fig. 7.16).

Post-operative recovery: within five days the whole surface of both cornea and conjunctiva had re-epithelialized and he was discharged home. Visual acuity one week post-operatively was 6/6 and has remained stable at this level (now two years post-operatively). His cornea cleared in the weeks after surgery (Figs 7.18 and 7.19). Note that the inferior fornix showed no evidence of symblepharon formation (Fig. 7.20).

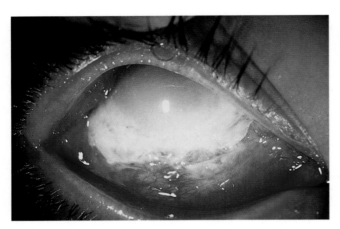

Figure 7.18. Post-operative picture showing the amniotic membrane in place.

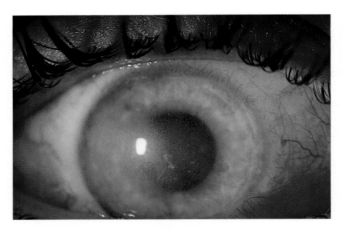

Figure 7.19. Three months later, the amniotic membrane is virtually absorbed. There is a faint superficial corneal haze.

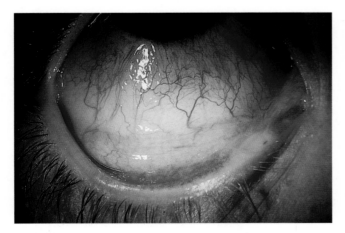

Figure 7.20. The same eye showing a normal inferior conjunctival fornix.

Limbal stem cell transplantation

Treatment of stem cell failure depends on whether the failure is partial/local or total/diffuse as well as whether the condition is unilateral or bilateral (see Figs 7.21a and b). In partial cases, the principle of treatment is to encourage the remaining stem cells to regenerate, and repopulate the cornea with normal epithelial cells. Local debridement of non-epithelialized cornea at the limbus may encourage circumferential migration of remaining limbal stem cells (LSCs). The presence of a layer of stem cells, no matter how thin, will prevent conjunctivalization of the cornea due to its barrier function. In cases where more than two clock-hours of stem cells have been lost, one can augment debridement with peritomy and use amniotic membrane as a bandage lens. Re-epithelialization can sometimes be achieved even with a small residual area of surviving stem cells with supportive measures to hold back advancing conjunctival-derived cells.

With more severe or total stem cell loss, there will be insufficient remaining LSC to maintain a normal stable corneal epithelium and recurrent erosions occur with a persistent epithelial defect resulting. LSC transplantation may be indicated.

The possible sources of these stem cells will depend on whether the underlying disease is unilateral or bilateral. Provided that there is no risk of developing the same condition in the fellow eye, the safest tissue to use for LSC transplant is stem cells from the fellow eye, i.e. limbal autografting (LAU). Taking up to four clock-hours of stem cells does not seem to lead to problems in the donor eye in unilateral cases. In bilateral conditions, of whatever cause, LSC autografting will not be an option, even if the involvement is very asymmetrical.

In these cases, limbal allografts (LALs) from a tissue-typed relative have been advocated. It is debatable whether this is any more advantageous than using cadaveric stem cells as immunosuppression is still going to be required (if not for the risk of rejection, it will be for the underlying disease state). It can also be difficult to find a relative who is a willing donor.

In allografting, systemic immunosuppression, e.g. with cyclosporin A, is essential although AMT is reputed to reduce the need for it. The duration of such treatment remains unclear but may well be lifelong. Careful counselling is needed, remembering that the side effects can be dangerous. Recruit the help of a physician experienced in immunosuppression.

It is essential to pre-screen the patient's renal (creatinine) and liver function and to measure the blood pressure. Start the treatment a week prior to surgery. The dose of Neoral (cyclosporin A) is 4–8 mg/kg of body weight. The dose is then usually reduced to 2–3 mg/kg of body weight and a serum trough level of 100–150 μg/l is aimed for. Monitoring of renal and liver functions and trough serum levels of cyclosporin A, as well as blood

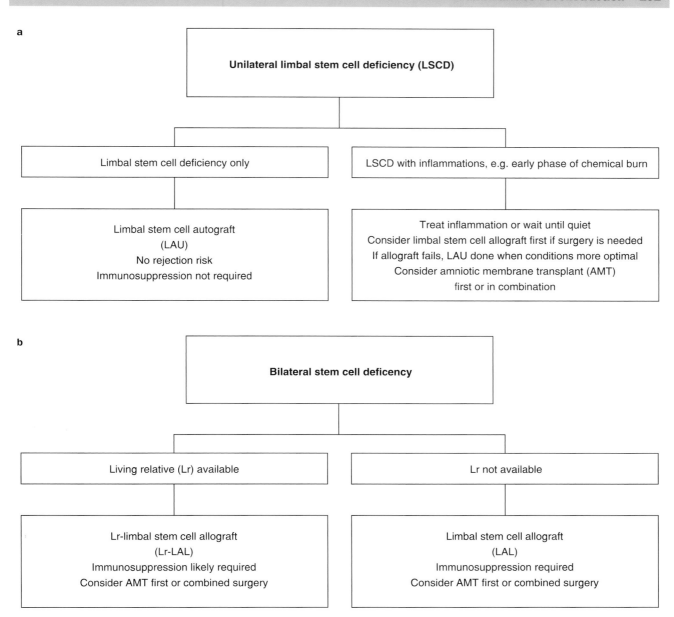

Figure 7.21. (a, b) Flow chart summarizing the treatment for unilateral and bilateral stem cell deficiency.

pressure, is then continued on a regular (monthly) basis. Record the creatinine level as a fraction of the baseline measurement, and do not allow the level of the creatinine to exceed 130 per cent of the starting level. For example if the baseline creatinine is 60 mg/l, a subsequent test result might be 74. Write this as 74/60, remembering the maximum will be 80/60. Higher levels indicate advancing renal failure.

Whereas autografts show greater than 90 per cent survival, the survival for LSC allografts has been reported as being between 70 per cent and 80 per cent in the first one to two years post-graft. By five years, survival is down to about 50 per cent (Table 7.17). Use of amniotic membrane during stem cell grafting has been shown to improve the prognosis.

The surgical techniques involved will now be described.

Table 7.17. Limbal allografts.

Success is defined as improvement in clinical picture.
Cyclosporin A or other immunosuppression required.
Augment treatment with autologous serum.
Survival, 70–80%, < 2 years.
Survival, ~ 50%, < 5 years.
Failure occurs when there is a recurrence of problems.
Causes of failure: allograft rejection, limbal inflammation.

TECHNIQUE FOR LIMBAL STEM CELL ALLOGRAFTING

Healthy limbal stem cells can be transferred to recipient corneas by using the peripheral corneoscleral tissue as the carrier (keratolimbal allografting or KLAL).

Anaesthesia

Either local or general anaesthesia may be used.

Preparing the recipient eye

Ensure adequate exposure of the eye. Use both superior and inferior rectus stay sutures (4-0 Prolene). If combining the procedure with penetrating keratoplasty, suture either a scleral-support band or Flieringa ring at the start of the procedure. A lateral canthotomy may also be required. Always prepare the recipient bed before starting on the donor dissection. These eyes invariably bleed, but if left alone, haemostasis will occur naturally and without any need to use cautery.

(1) Perform a 360 degree peritomy. A drop of phenyl-ephrine can reduce bleeding, but avoid using cautery unless the bleeding is torrential.

(2) A superficial keratectomy is done to denude the cornea of either abnormal epithelium or vascular pannus. Try to 'peel' this abnormal membrane off as a whole, and be wary of using sharp dissection if the cornea is very vascularized (see Fig. 7.22).

(3) Use the same size of trephine that will be used for the donor tissue and make a shallow cut into the cornea to receive the edge of the limbal graft.

Preparing the donor tissue

(1) Make a partial partial-thickness groove around the periphery of the donor cornea, using a trephine if more than a couple of clock-hours are to be used. Choose a trephine which is about 3 mm smaller than the corneal diameter.

(2) Cut a parallel incision in the scleral rim, about 2 mm peripheral to the limbus.

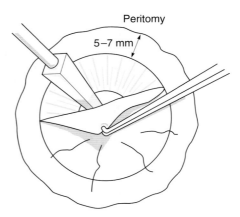

Figure 7.22. Preparing the recipient eye – debriding the fibrovascular pannus by 'peeling' it off the cornea as a whole piece.

(3) With a crescent blade knife, undercut this strip of tissue, cutting from the cornea towards the limbus. This creates a superficial lamellar circular strip of material that includes peripheral cornea, limbus and proximal sclera. Trim off any conjunctival tissue (see Fig. 7.23).

(4) If it is intended to transplant the cornea at the same time, trephine the corneal button and remove it to a

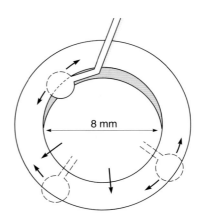

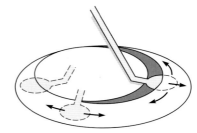

Figure 7.23. Preparing the donor tissue – using a circular blade to create a superficial lamellar flap of peripheral cornea, limbus, sclera and conjunctiva. The conjunctiva can be trimmed later.

watch-glass and cover with viscoelastic (Healon®) and BSS. The limbal tissues may then be dissected.

(5) The ring can be opened or further cut, making two segments; these are easier to suture into the donor bed. A gap will remain between the segments after suturing, but may be placed superiorly if there is functioning trabeculectomy.

(6) Two complete donor rings (i.e. two donor eyes) will be needed if one is to avoid any gaps through which growth of conjunctiva can still occur.

Transplanting the stem cells

(1) Place the anterior edge of the crescent or ring onto the host limbus in their correct anatomical orientation. Unless four crescents are available, there will invariably be a small gap left but this can be filled with donor tissue (e.g. corneal stroma). See Fig. 7.24.

(2) Using interrupted 10-0 vicryl or nylon, anchor the donor rim at corneal and then scleral margins.

(3) Make sure the corneal edge of the KLAL lies flush with recipient cornea.

(4) Ensure all the sutures are rotated and buried at the end of the procedure.

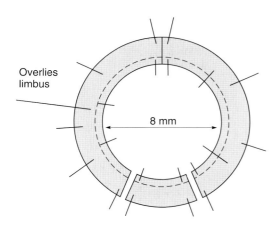

Overlies limbus

8 mm

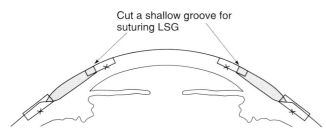

Cut a shallow groove for suturing LSG

Figure 7.24. Transplanting stem cells – placing the anterior edge of the crescent or ring onto the host limbus in the correct anatomical orientation. Suture the donor stem cells onto the recipient cornea starting with the donor and then the scleral rim.

(5) Cover with a contact lens or an amniotic membrane graft or both.

This method can be combined with an amniotic membrane transplant, a deep lamellar or a penetrating keratoplasty. Unless unavoidable, the corneal graft should be deferred until the ocular surface has been stable with functioning stem cells for at least three months. Otherwise, combining any corneal grafting with amniotic membrane transplantation is recommended.

Post-operative care

Topical treatment with preservative-free prednisolone 1 per cent and chloramphenicol (0.5 per cent) is used at least four times a day. This is then tapered off after one month. Systemic immunosuppression is required for allografts (as described above). Maintenance therapy includes topical steroids and systemic immunosuppression, which may be required lifelong even for living, related, HLA-matched donors.

TECHNIQUE FOR LIMBAL STEM CELL AUTOGRAFTING

It is vital to ensure that the fellow eye is not involved in the disease process before proceeding. If the process could possibly be bilateral (e.g. in a patient who has developed stem cell deficiency following a contact lens wear problem) an alternative approach must be used. Do not take more than four clock-hours of tissue in total. Avoid taking all the limbal tissue from the 12 and 6 o'clock positions where the stem cells are densest as this can lead to stem cell deficiency in the donor eye.

Anaesthesia

Use sub-Tenon's anaesthesia or general anaesthesia.

Instruments

Calipers, diamond knife (a front-running double-edged, calibrated diamond blade is recommended but is not essential), a disposable crescent blade, Micro grooved forceps, Micro needle holder, 10-0 vicryl suture.

Preparing the recipient bed

Avoid if possible disturbing the superior and inferior limbal zones, which even in depleted eyes may harbour a larger population of stem cells. Preparatory dissection is best done before tissue is harvested from the other eye. If this procedure is done in conjunction with a deep lamellar or penetrating keratoplasty, then a suitable scleral-support ring or a Flieringa ring may be sutured in place at this stage.

(1) Mark out the recipient beds. They may be located in either any area where there has obviously been a breakdown of the limbal barricade (e.g. pterygium), or based around 3 and 9 o'clock axes if there has been more generalized damage.

(2) The conjunctiva is recessed to about 5 mm from the limbus.

(3) Using the calibrated diamond knife set at 100 μm, make a superficial circumferential cut in the cornea and two radial incisions extending from the cornea to the sclera. The size marked out should be approximately two clock-hours and will match up to the donor slips that will be transferred. A crescent blade is used to dissect off a lamellar flap of cornea and create beds for the grafts. Any fibrovascular pannus is 'peeled' off as a whole if possible.

Avoid using cautery because of risk of causing further damage to the stem cells. When the tissue has been harvested from the fellow eye, it will be found that the bleeding will have stopped, and any clot can be easily wiped away. A drop of phenylephrine can also help reduce the bleeding.

Preparing the donor tissue

If treating a recurrent pterygium, donor tissue may be taken from the same eye and swung into place.

(1) Mark out, with partial-thickness radial incisions one or two, two clock-hour segments of limbus between 10 and 12 o'clock superiorly and 4 and 6 o'clock inferiorly. Extend these on to the sclera so that they are about 3 mm in length. The conjunctiva and episclera will bleed. Ignore this and it will stop without the need for cautery, which can damage the tissues that you are trying to transplant.

(2) Using the diamond knife, make shallow circumferential corneal incisions 1.5 mm inside the corneal limbus, extending between the radial cuts. This should be to an estimated depth of 150 μm.

(3) Make circumferential and parallel incisions in conjunctiva and sclera, thus marking the back of the donor patch.

(4) Use the crescent blade to carefully dissect this superficial lamella of cornea and limbus.

(5) Prior to cutting free this tiny fragment of tissue, insert one arm of the 10-0 vicryl through each corner of the corneal edge. This helps identify orientation and also gives a handle with which to move this tiny scrap of tissue (Fig. 7.25).

(6) Continue the dissection, shaving off the superficial sclera beyond the limbus and cut this free with a fringe of conjunctiva approximately 3 mm in length.

(7) Leave until the transplant is in place and only cauterize any bleeding points if bleeding persists.

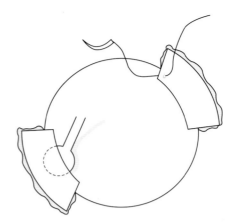

Figure 7.25. Mark out two clock-hour segments of peripheral cornea and limbus with partial-thickness radial incisions. Undercut this tissue with a crescent blade. Before removing it from the eye, place one anchoring 10-0 vicryl suture to help orientation.

The transplant

(1) Suture the donor tissue onto the recipient beds, using the sutures already in place. Take long bites to ease burying of the knots.

(2) Ensure that the patches are neatly fitting in the beds previously prepared.

(3) The donor and recipient conjunctiva are then sutured together using 10-0 vicryl (Fig. 7.26).

(4) Attempt to get the donor fragments gently stretched. This will make the graft smooth and more comfortable.

(5) A bandage contact lens is inserted into the recipient eye at the end of the procedure. Local anaesthetic and antibiotic ointment is instilled into the donor eye.

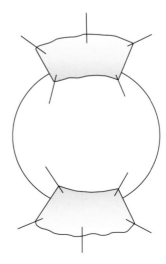

Figure 7.26. Suture the donor tissue with the preplaced sutures.

Worked Example 7.2: Chronic alkali burn treated with combined limbal stem cell and corneal auto-transplantation.

Case

A 67-year-old male had an alkali burn in his left eye in 1984. Although the eye was saved, the ocular surface was scarred and vascularized (Fig. 7.27). The surface was unstable and the vision poor at 6/36.

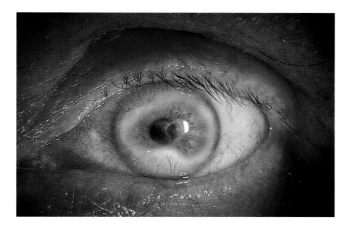

Figure 7.27. Appearance of the chemically-injured left eye four years post-injury.

Clinical findings

In May 1998, he presented to his optometrist complaining that the sight in his good right eye was misty. Examination showed that the sight of this eye was now less than 6/36 and ophthalmoscopy revealed a pigmented mass and he was referred for treatment (see Figs 7.28 and 7.29). A presumed diagnosis of

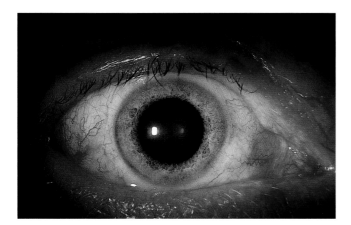

Figure 7.28. Normal looking anterior segment of the right eye.

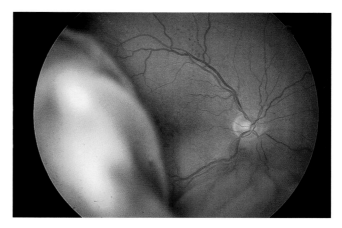

Figure 7.29. Fundus photograph showing a large choroidal melanoma in the right eye.

a choroidal melanoma was made and he was referred to an ocular oncologist for a second opinion regarding management of the eye.

CAT scanning suggested that there was trans-scleral spread of the tumour. After careful counselling he underwent enucleation of the tumorous eye and the left eye was prepared for reconstruction of the ocular surface and a corneal graft.

Operation

The recipient eye was prepared first by a partial-thickness trephination of 8.5 mm diameter. The peripheral pannus was removed and the conjunctiva recessed with a peritomy. The bleeding stopped naturally without the need for cautery.

An 8.5 mm vacuum trephine was used on the enucleated eye to mark out the inner margin of limbal tissue, cutting to approximately two-thirds depth. This 360 degree ring of tissue was carefully undermined (approximately 0.2 mm deep) with a crescent blade and freed. It was then transferred to the recipient eye. The trephination of the donor cornea was completed to remove the cornea, which was placed endothelial side up on a watch-glass covered with viscoelastic and BSS.

The limbal ring was opened and sutured in place using 10-0 vicryl.

The corneal graft was performed using 10-0 nylon. The eye was covered with a bandage contact lens and antibiotic drops instilled.

Post-operatively, dilute steroids and preservative-free antibiotic drops were given and the patient regularly reviewed. Three weeks post-operatively the visual acuity was 6/9 in this eye and the patient was able to function normally. He returned to work and driving. The eye remained stable, without recurrences of ocular surface problems, and treatment was stopped at six months (Fig. 7.30). All the sutures were removed at one year. Thirty months after surgery he developed secondary tumours from the melanoma from which he has succumbed.

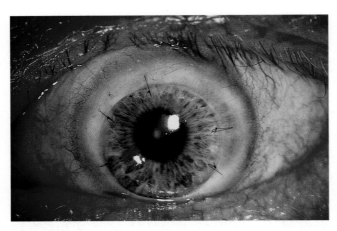

Figure 7.30. Appearance of the eye 18 months after surgery, showing a clear corneal graft supported by healthy stem cells.

Post-operative care

Preservative-free drops of prednisolone 0.5 per cent and chloramphenicol 0.5 per cent are given three times a day in the recipient eye. The donor eye is given either the same medication or chloramphenicol ointment. The treatment is extended for up to two weeks. Supplementary lubricants may also be needed. Re-epithelialization of the cornea should occur in about 10 days, at which stage the contact lens can be removed.

Conjunctival reconstruction

As mentioned previously, operations on the conjunctiva can lead to a more aggressive fibrotic reaction, especially when the disease is primarily autoimmune and careful thought is required before considering any surgical interference. In the acute situation, such as following a chemical injury, the potential for developing adhesions between the denuded bulbar and tarsal conjunctiva is great.

Different options have been advocated to prevent symblepharon formation, with variable successes. The regular sweeping of the fornices with glass rods in the early stages after an injury has been the treatment of choice to prevent adhesions, combined with gelatin sponges or a conformer. Lubricants and steroids are also needed. These techniques can also be used after dividing symblephara to prevent their reformation.

However, AMT has opened new hope in the treatment of these eyes, both in the acute and the chronic, reconstructive stages. The successful use of AMT to cover the surgically excised areas of symblepharon after chemical or thermal burns and Stevens–Johnson syndrome has been reported.

Nasal mucosa harvested from the middle turbinate bones has the added property of a very similar histology to normal conjunctiva with plentiful goblet cells. The tissue is sewn into the inferior fornix in a similar technique.

TECHNIQUE FOR CONJUNCTIVAL RECONSTRUCTION

Local or general anaesthesia can be used.

(1) Surgically remove the abnormal, scarred conjunctiva and subconjunctival fibrous tissue to expose healthy episclera or sclera.

(2) The entire area deficient of conjunctiva can be covered with amniotic membrane, *basement membrane surface up*. A conjunctival autograft, e.g. from the fellow eye (if normal), can also be used.

(3) Secure the membrane to the episclera just peripheral to the corneal limbus on one end and to residual conjunctival edge on the other end. Using interrupted 10-0 or 8-0 vicryl sutures.

(4) Place a symblepahron ring at the end of the procedure.

(5) If the fornix needs to be re-formed, do so by passing a set of double-armed 4-0 silk sutures through the conjunctiva (to the intended depth of the fornix), hitching into the periosteum of the orbital rim and exiting at the eyelid skin. Bolsters can be used to protect the skin.

(6) Post-operatively, topical steroids or combination drops such as maxitrol may be used in conjunction with lubricants, tapering the frequency over six to eight weeks.

Useful hints

(1) Irrigate continuously to wash blood away from the surgical field. Use wet-field cautery to achieve haemostasis.

(2) Phenylephrine 10 per cent, used either as a drop or on sponges soaked in the drug, can help reduce bleeding.

(3) The peritomy and conjunctival recession allows the remaining conjunctiva to retract, helping to create a new fornix, and clears the palpebral surface for AMT.

Deep lamellar or penetrating keratoplasty

Corneal surgery should be delayed until the other components of the ocular surface, e.g. lid position, tear film and stem cell population, have been properly addressed. If required, the surgery can be staged correcting one component at a time. Ideally, the eye should have been quiet for at least three months before deep lamellar or penetrating keratoplasty is considered. In severe ocular surface disease, not only will the limbal tissue and conjunctiva be severely affected, but these eyes will also have vascularized and deeply scarred corneas. These grafts are, without question, high-risk grafts. Use of amniotic membrane may help give added protection, but tissue-typed material and systemic immunosuppression must be considered and probably used. Sometimes, for instance if the cornea perforates, the situation will be forced and an emergency graft will be needed.

Provided that the existing OSD has been well managed (and probably if the disease is only mild or moderate), the result from corneal grafting can be quite good. Often however, particularly in the more damaged eyes, survival is poor and repeat grafts become necessary. The case for immunosuppression becomes more pressing.

Worked Example 7.3: Staged surgery – amniotic membrane transplantation followed by combined limbal stem cell allografting and penetrating keratoplasty in a case of severe acid injuries.

Case
This unfortunate tax inspector from Tanzania was assaulted with acid for refusing to take a bribe. He suffered severe burns to his eyes, face and trunk (Fig. 7.31). He had initial plastic surgery to his face there and was referred to the United Kingdom for ophthalmic and plastic surgical reconstruction.

Clinical findings
At presentation in the UK, horrific keloid scarring of his face, neck and upper trunk was noted. The eyelids were rigid and immobile (Fig. 7.32). The left eye was already blind and phthisical. His right eye could barely perceive light and slit-lamp

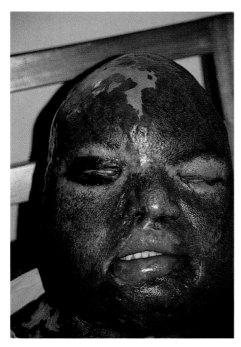

Figure 7.31. A photograph taken in the first 24 hours after the assault.

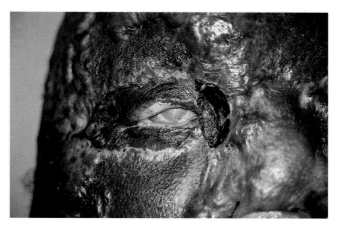

Figure 7.32. Photograph of the face showing keloid-scarred eyelids, opaque cornea and lagophthalmos.

examination showed a Hughes grade 4 chemical burn with total limbal stem cell loss. The cornea was vascularized and opaque with central thinning.

A multidisciplinary approach was needed with input from the anterior segment unit, the oculoplastics unit and the plastic surgeons. Ophthalmic interventions were aimed at attempting to refashion the eyelids to allow closure, and ocular surface reconstruction. A staged approach was necessary.

Surgery
Removal of keloids with full-thickness skin grafts. Plastic surgical repair of nose, ears and mouth was achieved. Free skin flaps were used and successfully released the rigid bars of keloid that prevented neck and jaw movements.

Ocular surface reconstruction
Stage 1: The corneal vascular pannus was removed and the cornea and conjunctiva were covered with a large amniotic membrane transplant. Six weeks post-operatively, he developed a descemetocele, necessitating an emergency corneal graft (Fig. 7.33).

Stage 2: He underwent a combined limbal stem cell allograft and penetrating keratoplasty. Immunosuppression with oral cyclosporin A (10 mg/kg/day) was commenced two days pre-operatively, and per-operatively he was given 500 mg of methylprednisolone intravenously.

Post-operative recovery

He developed a small leak in the graft–host interface, which required resuturing. The post-operative course was smoother after that. He was maintained on cyclosporin A and autolo-gous serum. At the time of his return to Tanzania six months after presentation, he had useful navigational (count fingers) vision in the right eye (see Fig. 7.34).

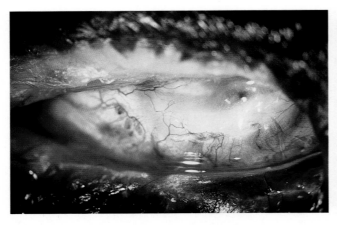

Figure 7.33. A descemetocele in his cornea, necessitating a corneal graft.

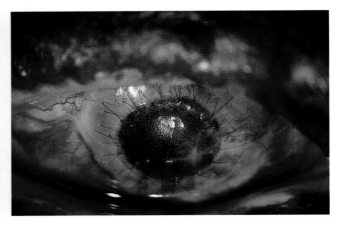

Figure 7.34. Appearance of the right eye following combined limbal stem cell allografting and penetrating keratoplasty – the cornea is reasonably clear with areas of normal corneal epithelium.

Where the disease is so extensive that reconstruction of the OS is impossible, a keratoprosthesis or a kerato-odonto-prosthesis may offer some hope for re-establishing vision.

Ocular surface reconstruction is a challenging new field with good successes described in the literature. However, since these are severely damaged eyes, the outcomes are often less than optimal and multiple surgeries are required. It is important therefore to establish a good relationship with the patient at the outset, as you will become well acquainted.

Section Four

Reparation and Rehabilitation

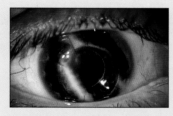

8 Evidence-based outcome measures following cataract and reconstructive surgery

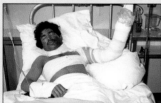

9 Medical jurisprudence for ophthalmologists

outcomes and complications if further intervention is needed. Certain key issues will be discussed.

Nd:YAG POSTERIOR LASER CAPSULOTOMY

The formation of significant posterior capsular opacification (PCO) can reduce the visual benefit of cataract surgery. A meta-analysis estimated the rate of PCO to be more than 25 per cent[8] after five years. However, the rate of laser capsulotomy is estimated to be falling to around 10 per cent[9]. This is due to several factors including better operative technique; PCO is known to be less if good cortical clearance is performed with an in-the-bag implant[10]. Other factors, such as biocompatibility (acrylic lenses better than unmodified polymethylmethacrylate [PMMA] and first-generation silicone lenses) and lens design (sharp, square-edged lenses have lower PCO), are also important[11]. To date, PCO is not preventable and laser capsulotomy with a Nd:YAG laser is required to restore vision. The problems this can cause are summarized in Table 8.5.

THE 'DROPPED' LENS FRAGMENT

One complication of phacoemulsification, which is rare in ECCE surgery, is the posterior dislocation of lens fragments, with an estimated incidence of 1.6 per 100,000[20]. With appropriate management, involving pars plana vitrectomy and lens fragment removal (if there is anything other than a quarter of the lens 'dropped' or if there is uncontrolled inflammation or glaucoma), the published results of the visual outcome are encouraging.

The timing for the referral is controversial, with studies suggesting no influence[20,21], or better outcome for early referral[22]. The chance of developing good vision ($\geq$6/12) and the risk of possible complications from the corrective vitreo-retinal surgery is summarized in Table 8.6.

The factors[20–22] associated with a poor visual outcome following vitrectomy and lensectomy/fragmentation are:

(1) Retinal detachment after surgery.
(2) Post-operative uveitis.
(3) Persistent cystoid macular oedema (CMO).
(4) Raised intraocular pressure (IOP).

Table 8.5. Dangers of Nd:YAG laser capsulotomy after cataract surgery.

Author	Type of complication	Incidence (%)
Ranta et al., 2000[12]	Retinal breaks	0.4
Olsen and Olson, 2000[13]	Retinal detachment (post ECCE)	3.1
	(post phaco)	0
Nissen et al., 1998[14]	Retinal detachment (myopic eyes)	6.0
Steinert et al., 1991[15]	Retinal detachment	0.89
Van Westenbrugge et al., 1992[16]	Retinal detachment	1.0
Ficker et al., 1987[17]	Retinal detachment	2.0
(AVERAGE)	Retinal detachment	(2.16%)
Olsen and Olson, 2000[13]	Cystoid macular oedema	0
Steinert et al., 1991[15]	Cystoid macular oedema	1.2
Albert et al., 1990[18]	Cystoid macular oedema	5.6
Lewis et al., 1987[19]	Cystoid macular oedema	0
(AVERAGE)	Cystoid macular oedema	(1.70%)
Steinert et al., 1991[15]	Worsening glaucoma	0.56

Table 8.6. Visual outcome and complications in patients treated for the posteriorly dislocated lens fragment.

Author	Visual outcome	Complications			Post-op
Uveitis	($\geq$6/12)	Retinal detachment		Raised IOP	CMO*
Watts et al., 2000[20]	83.3%	0%	11%	5.5%	11%
Bessant et al., 1998[22]	64.7%	18%	25%	32.5%	NR
Wong et al., 1997[23]	77.7%	27.7%	11.1%	NR	0%
Borne et al., 1996[21]	68%	16%	1.6%	3.3%	NR

* Cystoid macular oedema; NR = not recorded.

RETINAL DETACHMENT AFTER CATARACT SURGERY

Studies have suggested that there can be a 3.9[24] to 7.5[25] times higher risk of retinal detachment (RD) after cataract surgery than with no surgery. Table 8.7 gives the estimated risks for developing RD with the different techniques of cataract surgery. Phacoemulsification has been shown to have a low RD risk compared with the older techniques.

The risk factors for developing retinal detachment after cataract surgery are:

(1) Long/myopic axial length ($\geq$24 mm)[13,26]. Myopia is found in 40 per cent of patients with RD[27]. Patients with Stickler's syndrome run a 30 per cent risk of getting a RD[27]. Patients with Marfan's syndrome and homocystinuria also have a higher risk of developing retinal detachments after cataract surgery. The risks of retinal detachment in myopes after cataract surgery are between 0.3 per cent[28] to 2.0 per cent[14], but if combined with laser capsulotomy can be as high as 6 per cent[14].

(2) Posterior capsule rupture during cataract surgery[26].

(3) Nd:YAG laser capsulotomy[13,24,26].

(4) Ocular trauma after surgery[26].

(5) Type of surgery intracapsular cataract extraction (ICCE)>ECCE>phaco)[13].

(6) History of retinal detachment/lattice degeneration[26]. Lattice degeneration is found in up to 40 per cent of patients with retinal detachment[27]. However, the rate of RD in a population with lattice is approximately 0.06 per cent[29].

(7) Age $\leq$60 years[13].

(8) Male sex[13].

SECONDARY LENS IMPLANTATION, INCLUDING LENS EXCHANGE

Secondary IOL implantation offers an alternative to aphakic glasses or contact lenses in the visual rehabilitation of aphakia. Major implant-related complications although infrequent do occur, but in these patients a lens exchange is warranted since the patient initially expected the visual benefits of an IOL. However, in both these groups there is a significant rate of complications, which can result in visual loss in up to 29 per cent[30] of cases. The visual results from lens exchange are not unexpectedly poorer compared to secondary lens implantation[31] (see Table 8.8). The complications (Tables 8.9 and 8.10) can also be greater since lens exchange involves explanting the existing IOL and is usually done because of an ocular problem like cystoid macular oedema or persistent uveitis[30,31,40]. The risks must therefore be discussed fully with the patient beforehand.

Good visual results ($\geq$6/12) are achievable in a large proportion of cases using modern, anterior chamber (AC) IOLs, sulcus-fixated IOLs and sutured IOLs (iris-sutured or scleral-sutured). The information for secondary lens implantation and lens exchange has been grouped together because, on reviewing the literature, some of the papers did not separate the results between the two procedures, nor did they separate their results according to type of IOL used. The papers that were specific for each group or those that have a mix of results (termed 'mixed group') will be indicated in Tables 8.8 – 8.10, as will the type(s) of IOL used.

Anterior chamber intraocular lenses

The fourth-generation, flexible, open-looped AC IOLs with no holes remain a useful tool in treating aphakia. This applies not only in the developing world but also in certain clinical situations such as in secondary lens implantation, lens exchange and in complicated cataract cases (e.g. with capsular rupture without adequate capsular support). Their use requires good clinical judgement coupled with a good surgical technique. However, they are technically less demanding than performing sutured IOLs.

The efficacy of AC IOLs in primary cataract surgery has been proven in the developing world with two prospective, randomized clinical trials[44,45]. From these studies, an average of 93.4 per cent of patients achieved 6/12 or better vision, with complications occurring in 2.9 per cent of cases.

The use of modern, open-looped, AC IOLs for secondary lens implantation and lens exchange are well documented (see WE 8.2). The main concern in their use is the development of corneal decompensation, but the explantation rate has been reported as between 0.06 per cent and 0.16 per cent, five times lower than with closed-looped AC IOLs[46]. AC IOLs are associated with less serious complications, directly attributable to the IOL. In contrast, serious compli-

Table 8.7. Influence of type of cataract surgery on the development of retinal detachment.

Author	Intracapsular (ICCE)	Extracapsular (ECCE)	Phacoemulsification
Olsen and Olson, 2000[13]	5.4%	1.6%	0.4%
Norregaard et al., 1996[25]	NR	0.9%	NR
Tielsch et al., 1996[26]	NR	0.9%	NR
(AVERAGE)	NR	(1.1%)	NR

NR = not recorded.

Table 8.8. Visual expectations after secondary lens implantation/lens exchange.

Author (IOL type)	Post-operative vision			Visual loss
	≥6/12	6/15–6/36	≤6/60	
Open-loop AC IOL				
Kraff et al., 1983[32]	83%	N/A	N/A	5%
Ellerton et al., 1996[33]	85%	NR	NR	7.5%
(AVERAGE)	(84%)			(6.2%)
Iris-sutured PC IOL				
Navin-Aray, 1994[34]	63%	37%	0%	3.3%
Thompson and Noble (internal audit)[35]	69.2%	13.5%	17.3%	7.7%
(AVERAGE)	(66.1%)	(25.2%)	(8.6%)	(5.5%)
Scleral-sutured PC IOL				
Price and Wellemeyer, 1995[36]	84%	10.5%	5.3%	NR
McCluskey and Harrisberg, 1994[37]	75%	8.3%	16.7%	0%
Lewis, 1993[38]				
(Scleral-sutured + flap)	57%	NR	NR	10%
(Scleral-sutured, no flap)	63%	NR	NR	2.5%
(AVERAGE)	(69.8%)	(9.4%)	(11%)	(4.2%)
Mixed group				
Price and Wellemeyer 1995[36] (scleral-sutured)	61.6%	21.7%	16.7%	21%
Hayward et al., 1990[39] (open-loop AC/PC IOL)	60%	21%	10%	23%
Stark et al., 1989[31] (scleral/iris-sutured)	100%	0%	0%	0%
(AVERAGE)	(73.9%)	(14.2%)	(8.9%)	(14.7%)
Lens exchange				
Pande and Noble, 1993*[40] (AC/sulcus support/PC IOL)	77%	13%	10%	7%
Coli et al., 1993*[30] (Iris/scleral-sutured/sulcus support)	49%	35%	6%	29%
Stark et al., 1989*[31] (Scleral/iris-sutured)	50%	50%	0%	12.5%
(AVERAGE)	(58.7%)	(32.7%)	(5.3%)	(16.2%)

*Lens exchange (note that the visual outcome in this group is not as good as for secondary IOLs); NR = not recorded; N/A = not applicable.

Worked Example 8.2

Case
A 42-year-old surveyor presented in 1982, 10 years after blunt injury to the right eye which had caused iris loss and a traumatic cataract.

Clinical findings
Visual acuity: hand movement right and 6/9 corrected left. He had a stony hard cataract (Fig. 8.3), which was removed with the ocutome and an anterior chamber lens implanted.

Outcome
VA of 6/9 right and left 18 years after reconstruction (See Fig. 8.4 on following page).

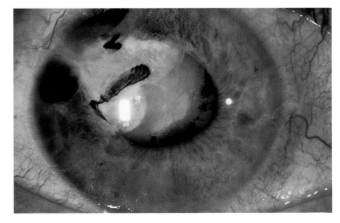

Figure 8.3. Traumatic cataract following a blunt injury.

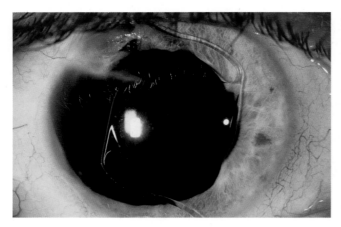

Figure 8.4. Post-operative picture of the same eye as Fig. 8.3, showing a well-positioned AC IOL.

cations like retinal detachment have been reported with sutured IOLs (particularly scleral-sutured IOLs), these being linked with imperfect surgical technique[47]. Inaccurate sizing of the AC IOL can lead to problems (see WE 8.3).

Sutured posterior chamber intraocular lenses

Sutured posterior chamber IOLs provide better optical and anatomical placement of IOLs than AC IOLs in eyes without capsular support. They are particularly useful in eyes with AC angle abnormalities and when the AC is shallow. On the whole, sutured PC IOLs are associated with a lower rate of corneal problems, iritis and glaucoma than AC IOLs [43,46,48]. However, sutured PC IOLs require greater surgical skill to implant and can also lead to more serious complications.

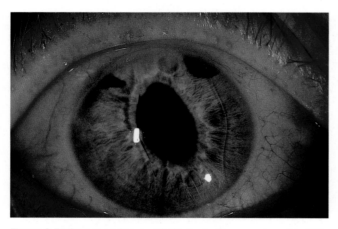

Figure 8.5. Over-sized Choyce AC IOL leading to an oval pupil in WE 8.3.

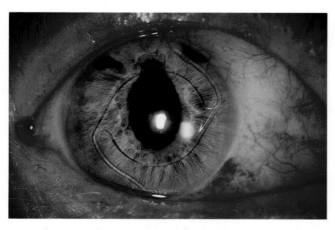

Figure 8.6. Relief of iris traction following lens exchange.

Worked Example 8.3

Case
An 87-year-old professor's wife had an uncomplicated intra-capsular cataract extraction in 1980 with implantation of a Choyce AC IOL.

Clinical findings
Vision of 6/36. Very tender eye to the touch. Clear cornea, but a low-grade uveitis and IOP of 25 mmHg. Vertically oval pupil due to an over-sized lens with iris capture (Fig. 8.5). There was also vitreous incarceration in the wound. Cystoid macular oedema, accounted for the reduced vision.

Reconstruction
Pre-treatment with topical steroids for two months prior to surgery. Supero-temporal incision, away from the primary wound site. Choyce IOL rotated out of the eye. Anterior vitrectomy done carefully, clearing strands from the anterior surface of the iris. Implantation of a replacement AC lens and continuous suture to the wound.

Outcome
Pain-free, with a vision of 6/18 at 12 months post-op. IOP was 14 mmHg (Fig. 8.6). The patient was delighted with the comfort and improved vision.

Learning points
(i) Too large an AC IOL and iris entrapment can lead to a low-grade uveitis, glaucoma and chronic pain.
(ii) Exchange of the lens usually removes the discomfort and may lead to improvement in vision.

Table 8.9. Incidence of sight-threatening complications after secondary lens implantation/lens exchange.

Author	Type		
	Retinal detachment	**Endophthalmitis**	**Corneal decompensation**
Open-loop AC IOL			
Ellerton et al., 1996[33]	1.2%	0%	1.2%
Weene, 1993[41]	0%	0%	11.6%
Kraff et al., 1983[32]	1.5%	0%	0%
(AVERAGE)	(0.9%)	(0%)	(4.3%)
Iris-sutured PC IOL			
Navin-Aray, 1994[34]	0%	0%	0%
Thompson et al.[*35]	5.7%	1.9%	11%
(AVERAGE)	(2.8%)	(1.0%)	(5.5%)
Scleral-sutured PC IOL			
Bourke et al., 1996[42]	8%	NR	NR
McCluskey and Harrisberg, 1994[37]	3.1%	0%	0%
(AVERAGE)	(5.5%)		
Mixed group			
Price and Wellemeyer 1995[36]	0%	0%	26%
Hayward et al., 1990[39]	2%	0%	2%
(AVERAGE)	(1%)	(0%)	(14%)
Lens exchange			
Pande and Noble, 1993[40]	3%	0%	6.6%
Coli et al., 1993[30]	2%	0%	23.5%
(AVERAGE)	(2.5%)	(0%)	(15%)

* Internal audit; NR = not recorded.

Worked Example 8.4

Case
A 50-year-old woman with megalocornea and myopia presented for cataract surgery. A routine lens was implanted and disappeared into the capsule and was retrieved. A large 14 mm lens was then tried which also sank inferiorly and was also removed. An iris-sutured technique was then used to maintain the central position of the lens.

Outcome
VA of 6/6 with +1.50 dioptres-sphere correction (Fig 8.7).

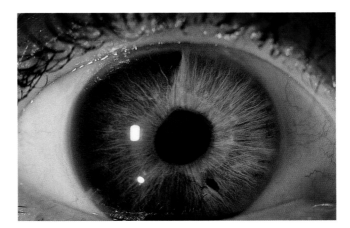

Figure 8.7. Two 'snake-bite' iridotomies can be seen in relation to the iris sutures with slight ovalling superiorly of the pupil. The lens is stable with normal IOP.

(1) Iris-sutured PC IOLs
In the only randomized, prospective study, by Schein et al.[49], iris-sutured PC IOLS were associated with the least complications. They provide good lens centration and are safer to use than when a trans-scleral approach is required, with mainly pupil distortion and iris transillumination being reported (see WE 8.4). When combined with penetrating keratoplasty, the 'open-sky' technique simplifies this approach.

(2) Scleral-sutured PC IOLs
When there is inadequate iris support, AC IOLs and iris-sutured IOLs cannot be used and this is where a trans-scleral approach becomes useful. This technique is, however, associated with more complications including sight-

Table 8.10. Incidence of other complications of secondary lens implantation/lens exchange

Author	Type (%)			
	CMO	Glaucoma (new/worse)	Corneal infection	Other
AC IOL				
Ellerton et al., 1996[33]	1.2%	0%	0%	N/A
Weene, 1993[41]	2.3%	0%	0%	N/A
Kraff et al., 1983[32]	NR	NR	0.5%	N/A
(AVERAGE)	(1.8%)	(0%)	(0.17%)	
Iris-sutured IOL				
Navin-Aray, 1994[34]	3.3%	13.3%	0%	N/A
Thompson et al.*[35]	11%	9.6%	0%	5.8% (lens decentration)
(AVERAGE)	(7.2%)	(11.4%)	(0%)	
Scleral-sutured				
Solomon et al., 1993[43]	0%	0%	0%	73% (suture erosion)
				10% (lens decentration)
Lewis, 1993[38]	19%	16%	10%	20% (flap suture erosion)
(AVERAGE)	(9.5%)	(8%)	(5%)	
Mixed goup				
Price and Wellemeyer 1995[36]	0%	9.3%	0%	13.3% (bleed)
				1.3% (lens dislocated)
Hayward et al., 1990[39]	15%	2%	0%	0%
(AVERAGE)	(7.5%)	(5.6%)	(0%)	
Lens exchange				
Pande and Noble, 1993[40]	10%	0%	0%	0%
Coli et al., 1993[30]	N/A	2.9%	0%	0%
(AVERAGE)		(1.4%)	(0%)	

*Internal audit; N/A = not applicable.

threatening retinal detachment and vitreous haemorrhage[42,43,49]. It was reported that 75 per cent of cases of RD in scleral-sutured IOLs were associated with vitreous incarceration by the intraocular suture[42].

The placing of the point of the needle penetration, and control of the position of the haptics of the IOL, can be made more precise using an ocular endoscope[50].

The visual outcome from secondary lens implantation and lens exchange are summarized in Table 8.8. The incidence and type of complications in these procedures are shown in Tables 8.9 and 8.10.

PENETRATING KERATOPLASTY

Setting the standards

From collective studies, the best outcome from penetrating keratoplasty (PKP) are those done for keratoconus. The Australian Corneal Graft Registry[51] (ACGR), with the largest amount of prospectively collected information on corneal grafts, reported a better than 95 per cent, 10-year survival in this group when the operation was performed by the 'frequent' grafter (more than 40 grafts per year). The

survival was down to 87.3 per cent for this period when surgery was performed by the 'occasional' grafter, doing less than 10 grafts per year. In terms of visual outcome, 78 per cent of grafts performed for keratoconus achieved a post-graft vision of $\geq 6/12$ with only 8 per cent of cases not gaining or losing vision. The authors' own internal audit[52] on PKPs reflected this outcome, with an over 95 per cent 10-year survival in grafts done for keratoconus. The outcome of all other PKPs should therefore be compared against the standards set by grafts done for keratoconus.

The reasons for graft failure are summarized in Table 8.11. Graft rejection remains the main cause of failure.

Poor prognostic indicators for graft survival

In general, the poor prognostic indicators[51,54–57] for graft survival are:

(1) The Centre effect: Surgeons doing less than 10 grafts per year (the 'occasional' grafter) have poorer results than those who perform more than 40 grafts per year (the 'frequent' grafter).

Table 8.11. Reasons for corneal graft failure.

Reasons for graft failure	Burr and Noble (internal audit)[52]	ACGR, 1996[51]	Kirkness et al., 1990[53] (repeat grafts)
Graft rejection	28%	32%	48%
Perforation	20%	2%	NR
Infection	16%	14%	9%
Corneal decompensation	11%	NR	15%
Primary failure	9%	5%	4%
Ocular trauma	6%	2%	NR
Recurrence of disease	1%	NR	17%
Glaucoma	0%	8%	0% (but 38% glaucoma prevalence)

NR = not recorded.

(2) Past inflammation.

(3) Deep vascularization of the recipient cornea.

(4) History of raised IOP/glaucoma.

(5) Presence of an AC IOL or iris-clip lens.

(6) Grafts done for primary endothelial failure.

(7) Graft size ≥ 8 mm.

(8) Patient age <10 years.

The risk factors for graft rejection[55] are:

(1) Mixed sutures.

(2) Larger grafts.

(3) Poor HLA Class I matching.

(4) Zero HLA-DR mismatching.

Penetrating keratoplasty for aphakic or pseudophakic bullous keratopathy

A significant proportion of corneal grafts are done for pseudophakic (PBK) or aphakic (ABK) bullous keratopathy. From the United Kingdom Transplant Study[58] and the ACGR[51], an average of 24 per cent of all corneal grafts were done for this problem. The survival (Table 8.12) and visual results of corneal grafting for bullous keratopathy are significantly worse compared with the 'standard' of keratoconus, e.g. overall graft 10-year graft survival for ABK/PBK is 47 per cent compared to over 95 per cent for keratoconus.

The visual outcome for bullous keratopathy is also less good when compared to corneal decompensation from Fuchs' endothelial dystrophy (Table 8.13). This reflects

Table 8.12. Corneal graft survival – comparing keratoconus with aphakic/pseudophakic bullous (ABK/PBK) keratopathy.

Authors	2-year	5-year	10-year
Australian Corneal Graft Registry, 1996[51]			
Keratoconus			
Occasional grafter	NR	97.9%	87.3%
Frequent grafter		98.1%	98.1%
Aphakic BK	NR	55.4%	37.8%
Pseudophakic BK	NR	57.3%	20.8%
Burr and Noble*[52]			
Keratoconus	95.1%	95.1%	95.1%
Aphakic BK	NR	NR	55%
Pseudophakic BK	NR	NR	75%
Other studies on bullous keratopathy			
Volker-Dieben et al., 1982[59]	60%	NR	NR
Bishop et al., 1986[60]	85%	50%	NR
Sugar, 1989[61]	83%	65%	NR
(AVERAGE for keratoconus (frequent grafter))		(96.6%)	(96.6%)
(AVERAGE for BK)	76%	56.9%	47.2%

* Internal audit; NR = not recorded.

Table 8.13. Visual outcome following corneal grafts – comparing keratoconus, Fuchs' endothelial dystrophy and aphakic/pseudophakic bullous (ABK/PBK) keratopathy.

Authors	≥6/12	6/18–6/60	≤6/60
Australian Corneal Graft Registry, 1996[51]			
Diagnosis			
Keratoconus	78%	12.6%	9.4%
Fuchs' endothelial dystrophy	51%	30%	19%
Pseudophakic bullous keratopathy	18%	32%	50%
Aphakic bullous keratopathy	19%	31%	50%
Burr and Noble*[52]			
Diagnosis			
Keratoconus	86%	11%	3%
Fuchs' endothelial dystrophy	77%	11%	11%
Pseudophakic bullous keratopathy	25%	50%	25%
Aphakic bullous keratopathy	33%	11%	56%
Other studies			
Olson et al., 1979[62] (ABK)	14.3%	14.3%	52.4%

*Internal audit; NR = not recorded.

on the damage caused from surgical complications, highlighting once again, not only the importance of avoiding complications during cataract surgery but in adequately handling the complications when they do occur. When PKP is required, it is best done or referred to the 'frequent' grafter for optimal results.

Lens-related procedures

Lens-related procedures take place in up to 27 per cent of PKPs[51]. Patients who have an IOL inserted or exchanged at time of grafting have a better graft survival than those retaining an existing IOL (usually iris-clip or older style IOL) or who remain aphakic, with a 10-year survival of 51.5 per cent compared to 27.3 per cent and 32.3 per cent, respectively[51]. The results from the ACGR, looking at specific lens types, are summarized in Table 8.14 and it

Table 8.14 Comparison of corneal graft survival rates with the different IOL types (from the Australian Corneal Graft Registry).

Lens type	1-year	5-year	8-9 year
PC IOL	91.5%	71.5%	60.5%
Sutured PC IOL	92.0%	73.3%	NR
AC IOL at PKP	92.4%	56.4%	43%
Pre-graft AC IOL	86.5%	32.6%	32.6%
Iris AC IOL	75.1%	30.3%	17.7%

NR = not recorded.

shows that PC IOLs fare best, highlighting the advantage of placing the IOL in a more natural anatomical position. Another important finding was that performing a simultaneous triple procedure rather than staging the lens and corneal graft procedure does not seem to lead to a worse outcome.

Penetrating keratoplasty with secondary lens implantation/lens exchange

With the available techniques of suturing IOLs, be it scleral or iris-sutured, there is little reason in leaving a patient aphakic and requiring high-powered contact lenses or glasses for visual rehabilitation. The quality of vision is going to be greater if the eye is not left aphakic.

It is accepted that sutured PC IOLs are technically more demanding but is made easier when done together with a corneal graft. However, there are studies showing that a post-operative visual acuity of ≥6/12 is achievable in between 57 to 75 per cent of eyes following PKP and an open-loop (e.g. the Kelman-style) anterior chamber IOL with ≥95 per cent graft survival in the study period[63,64]. Every effort should therefore be made to ensure that eyes requiring PKP for aphakia or bullous keratopathy have an IOL, unless it is unnecessary to do so, e.g. high myopia or in eyes with poor visual potential. Tables 8.15 and 8.16 summarize the visual outcome and complications seen in PKPs with secondary lens implantation/lens exchange.

Table 8.15. Visual expectations after corneal grafts with secondary lens implantation/lens exchange.

Author and IOL type		Post-operative vision		
	Follow-up	⩾6/12	6/15–6/36	⩽6/60
Open-loop AC IOL				
Schein et al., 1993[49]	18 months	18.2%	33.3%	46.9%
Hassan et al., 1991[63]	1 year	39.3%	NR	NR
	2 years	63.2%	NR	NR
	3 years	63.6%	NR	NR
Iris-sutured PC IOLs				
Schein et al., 1993[49]	18 months	31%	41.4%	27.6%
Hassan et al., 1991[63]	1 year	45.1%	NR	NR
	2 years	63.6%	NR	NR
Soong et al., 1989[65]	1 year	45.1%	30.5%	24.4%
	2 years	63.6%	18.2%	18.2%
Scleral-fixated				
Schein et al., 1993[49]	18 months	26.3%	42.1%	31.6%

NR = not recorded.

Table 8.16. Incidence of complications in corneal grafts with secondary lens implantation/lens exchange.

Type of Complication		Hassan et al.[63] AC IOL (iris-sutured)	Soong et al. [65] Iris-sutured
		Incidence	
	Sight-threatening		
2.3%	Retinal detachment	2.5% (2.3%)	
1.5%	Endophthalmitis	0%	
	Others		
	Cystoid macular oedema	32.5% (36.1%)	
36.4%	Glaucoma	22.5% (36.4%)	

OCULAR TRAUMA

The yearly cumulative incidence of ocular trauma requiring hospital admission is estimated to be 8.14 per 100,000 of the population in the UK[66]. The incidence of penetrating ocular injury itself is predicted to be about 3.6 per 100,000 of the population (Australian study)[67]. Up to 236 patients per year can expect to be permanently blinded in the injured eye, in the UK[66]. In the paediatric age group, the yearly cumulative incidence of ocular trauma is slightly higher than for the rest of the population at 8.85 per 100,000 in the UK[68]. The commonest place where ocular trauma, including blinding injury, occurs is the home (>50 per cent), in both adults[66,69] and children[68]. Assault accounts for up to 16.2 per cent of eye injuries in adults[69] and 14 per cent in children[68]. The implementation of good health and safety strategies are likely to reduce the frequency of these injuries.

Visual outcome following ocular trauma

The visual outcome following any type of ocular trauma appears favourable, with 86.8 per cent of adults[66] and 98 per cent of children recovering to 6/12[68] or better. The same studies[66,68] showed that severe visual loss (<6/60) was more common in adults (10.7 per cent) than in children (1 per cent).

The factors[70,71] that correlate to a favourable (>6/18) visual outcome are:

(1) Initial visual acuity at presentation of ≥6/60.
(2) Absence of an afferent pupillary defect.
(3) Location of wound anterior to the pars plana.
(4) Size of wound ≤10 mm.
(5) Sharp injury.

Factors[71] associated with a poor (<6/60 or 5/200) visual outcome include:

(1) Initial visual acuity <6/60 (5/200).
(2) Presence of an afferent pupillary defect.
(3) Blunt injury causing globe rupture.
(4) Wounds involving the sclera and/or extending posterior to the rectus muscle insertions.
(5) Size of wound >10 mm.
(6) Subluxed lens or when the lens is lost through the wound.
(7) A vitreous haemorrhage sufficient enough to obscure the view of the posterior segment.

Penetrating keratoplasty for ocular trauma

From the UKTS study of 1993[58], 3.2 per cent of corneal grafts were done for ocular trauma. Up to 34 per cent of corneal grafts repeated were because of trauma to the grafted eye. The 1–2-year graft survival rate and the visual outcomes (Table 8.17) following PKP for trauma, like those done for bullous keratopathy, fall short of those done for keratoconus (Table 8.13). Both these groups represent damaged eyes, the former from accident or assault and the latter from a surgical complication. The complications of PKP done for trauma are summarized in Table 8.18.

The poor prognostic indicators for graft survival following trauma are:

(1) Timing: Nobe et al.[76] showed that following corneal perforations for trauma, delaying PK for at least three months resulted in a better rate of graft clarity (80 per cent compared to 50 per cent).

Other indicators[77] for a poor outcome were:

(2) Blunt injury, as opposed to a small sharp penetrating injury.

(3) Initial laceration involving >10 mm of cornea or involving the sclera.

(4) Presence of posterior segment injury, e.g. retinal detachment, vitreous bleed or uveal prolapse.

Rotational grafts have a higher rate of survival, even those associated with the more advanced lens fixation techniques (see WE 8.5).

Penetrating keratoplasty for trauma in children

As for adults, PKP performed for ocular trauma can have a less favourable visual outcome compared to the standard (keratoconus). However, a significant percentage do get

Table 8.17. Graft survival and visual outcomes after penetrating keratoplasty for trauma.

Authors	Cases	Graft survival	Post-op. vision (improvement)	Study period (mean months)
Adults				
Doren et al., 1990[72]	41	80%	74%, ⩾ 6/30 (82%, vision improved)	12
Kenyon et al., 1992[73]	39	80%	49%, ⩾ 6/30 (72%, vision improved)	23
(AVERAGE)		(80%)	(77%, vision improved)	
Children				
Dana et al., 1995[74]	25	84% 70%	(83% vision improved)	12 24
Doren et al., 1990[72]	8	62%	NR	12
Stulting et al., 1984[75]	31	70%	17%, ⩾ 6/12 (87%, vision improved)	12
(AVERAGE)		(72%)	(85%, vision improved)	

Table 8.18. Complications of penetrating keratoplasty for trauma.

Complications	Authors			
	Doren et al., 1990[72]	Kenyon et al., 1992[73]	Dana et al., 1995[74]	Average
Secondary glaucoma	31%	46%	18%	32%
Rejection	25%	NR	36%	31%
Retinal detachment	8%	2.5%	4%	4.8%
Endophthalmitis	2.5%	0%	0%	0.8%

NR = not recorded.

Worked Example 8.5

Case
A 33-year-old agricultural worker was under a tractor, chipping rust from the exhaust, when the chisel he was using fell, blade first, into his left eye.

Clinical findings
He presented three years after the original injury with visions of 6/6 right and counting finger (CF) left. The eye was quiet but had extensive fibrosis of the remaining lens capsule. There was an oblique corneal scar running through the visual axis (Fig. 8.8).

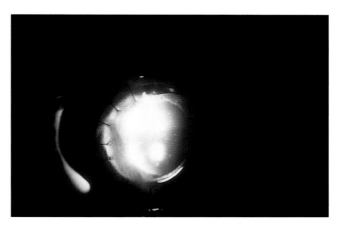

Figure 8.9. Red-reflex photograph showing the Morcher lens *in situ*.

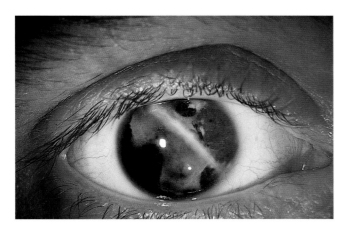

Figure 8.8. Linear corneal scar and dense membrane.

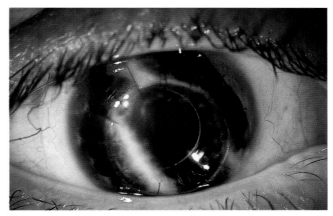

Figure 8.10. Completion of the rotational autograft, with clear cornea in the visual axis.

Reconstruction
An eccentric corneal button was cut, allowing access to the anterior chamber. The membrane and residual capsule were carefully dissected away. This left an obvious iris defect. A Morcher artificial pupil lens was fixated to the sclera (Fig. 8.9) and the corneal button was replaced, having been rotated by 180 degrees. This allowed clear cornea to be centred on the visual axis (Fig. 8.10).

Outcome
Post-operative vision was 6/6-2 unaided at two years.

Learning points
(i) A linear corneal scar running through the visual axis can be managed with a rotational autograft.
(ii) An artificial-pupil IOL can reduce the glare and photophobia associated with large iris defects.

---

visual improvement (see Table 8.17). As for traumatic cataracts, compliance with refractive aids required for improving vision (and treating amblyopia) can be problematic.

The poor prognostic indicators[75] for PKP following trauma in children are:

(1) If vitrectomy is required – suggesting mid/posterior segment injury.
(2) Pre-operative vascularization in the cornea.
(3) Presence of a persistent epithelial defect.

TRAUMATIC CATARACTS IN CHILDREN

As discussed in the Paediatrics chapter (Chapter 6), cataract surgery in this age group presents a greater challenge in terms of technique, choice of implant (or no implant) and post-operative inflammatory response. Children up to the age of nine years and perhaps older, face the additional risk of developing amblyopia and this can be a cause of poor visual outcome despite technically sound surgery. The visual outcome following traumatic cataract surgery is summarized in Table 8.19, while Table 8.20 reveals the possible complications.

The poor prognostic indicators are:

(1) Presence of ocular co-morbidity[80].
(2) Complex trauma, involving mid/posterior segment[78].
(3) Delay in referral for lensectomy[78].
(4) Inadequate treatment for post-operative aphakia, e.g. contact lens problems[78,80].
(5) Poor compliance with amblyopia therapy[78].

ACUTE SUPRACHOROIDAL HAEMORRHAGE

This potentially devastating complication is associated with various intraocular procedures including routine cataract surgery, glaucoma filtration surgery and penetrating keratoplasty. The use of smaller, self-sealing incisions with phacoemulsification has led to suprachoroidal haemorrhages being more limited and non-expulsive. Suprachoroidal haemorrhage is a potentially serious complica-

tion when doing scleral-sutured IOL, occurring in 3 per cent of cases[43]. The incidence of suprachoroidal haemorrhage during cataract surgery is shown in Table 8.21.

The risk factors[81,82] associated with this complication in cataract surgery are:

(1) Posterior capsular rupture with vitreous loss during surgery.
(2) Long axial length (myopia).
(3) Glaucoma.
(4) Atherosclerosis.
(5) Hypertension.
(6) Diabetes mellitus.
(7) Older age.
(8) Per-operative tachycardia.
(9) Excessive volume anaesthetic.
(10) Adrenaline use in retrobulbar anaesthetic.

The incidence and risk factors for acute suprachoroidal haemorrhage are summarized in Table 8.21.

END NOTE

The impact of trauma and the benefits of repair are not easily quantifiable for these damaged patients. The success and failure rates for each operation are important justifications for intervention, but do not convey the human price of the injury. Litigation may provide a financial recompense, but the effect on life-style – employment, economics of their family unit, loss of confidence – exerts a higher price than any monetary compensation can provide.

Table 8.19. Visual expectations after traumatic cataract surgery in children.

Author	⩾6/12	6/15–6/60	<6/60	Lost vision
Churchill et al., 1995[78]	59%	19%	22%	6%
Eckstein et al., 1998[79]	67%	29%	4%	0%
Hiles, 1984[80]	60%	14%	26%	NR

NR = not recorded.

Table 8.20. Complications from traumatic cataract surgery in children.

Author	Endophthalmitis	Retinal detachment	Others
Churchill et al., 1995*[78]	6%	9%	25% (squint)
Hiles, 1984[80]	0%	1%	18% (squint)
Eckstein et al., 1998[79]	0%	0%	19% (severe uveitis) 92% (PC opacity)
(AVERAGE)	(2%)	(3.3%)	

* Results reflect smaller numbers and differing complexity of cases.

Table 8.21. Incidence of suprachoroidal/expulsive haemorrhage in cataract surgery and other types of surgery.

Type of surgery	Incidence (%)	Risk factors
Cataract surgery		
Extracapsular cataract (ECCE)	0.13%[24]	See text
	0.16%[70]	
(AVERAGE)	(0.14%)	
Phacoemulsification	0.03%[24]	See text
Glaucoma filtration		
Givens and Shields, 1987[83]		As for cataract surgery, plus
Overall incidence	1.6%	Aphakia
If past vitrectomy	13%	Past vitrectomy
If aphakic and past vitrectomy	33%	
Speaker et al., 1991[82]		
Overall incidence	0.15%	
(AVERAGE overall incidence)	(0.88%)	
Penetrating keratoplasty		
Speaker et al., 1991[82]	0.56%	As for cataract surgery, plus
Price et al., 1994[84]	0.45%	Past vitrectomy (with A/C IOL)
(AVERAGE)	(0.55%)	
Vitreo-retinal procedures		
Speaker et al., 1991[82]	0.14%	As for cataract surgery

Worked Example 8.6

Case
A 35-year-old male had suffered an injury at work leaving him with very little sight in his right eye. The eye was intensely painful and so severe that he was not able to sleep and had lost his job. Three years after the injury he was referred for consideration for surgical reconstruction.

Clinical findings
Patient appeared in poor health, unshaven and in pain (Fig. 8.11a). Right eye divergent, ptosis, visual acuity of perception of light (PL), good projection; globe exquisitely tender; no relative afferent pupillary defect (RAPD); IOP normal at 16 mmHg.

Slit-lamp
Findings showed the presence of ¼ segment of corneal scar and general corneal haze, cataract, 2+ uveitis (Fig. 8.11b).

Management
The possible treatment was discussed with the patient. He was given frequent topical steroid drops for six weeks and at review the eye was quiet and the general corneal haze had cleared. It was felt that there was too much inflammation to do a penetrating corneal allograft and a rotational graft was suggested as a temporizing measure.

Operation
Right rotating corneal autograft, lensectomy, partial pupil repair, AC IOL implantation; botulinum toxin injected into the lateral rectus muscle at the end of surgery.

Post-operative progress
Post-operatively, the eye was quiet and the vision recovered rapidly. Topical steroids were maintained, but on a reducing frequency and strength over the 12 months after surgery. He was then maintained on daily steroid drops for three years. At the end of the first year he had returned to work and was now sleeping normally and looking forward to promotion at work. The improvement in his general appearance is dramatic (Fig. 8.11c).

Findings at 12 months
Slit-lamp appearance shows the dramatic clearing of the cornea and in particular the segment of inflamed cornea that had been rotated away. The visual acuity was measured at 6/9 uncorrected, 6/6 corrected. The IOP was normal and the eye quiet (Fig. 8.11d).

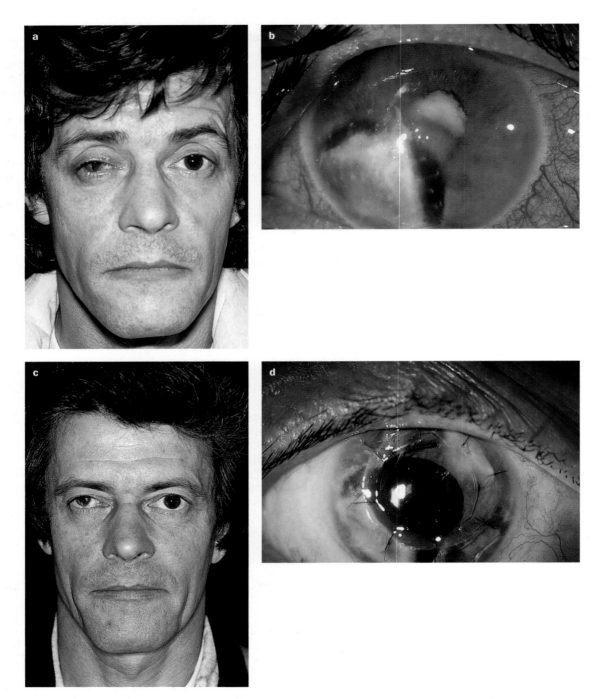

Figure 8.11. (a) Full face showing appearance at presentation. (b) Appearance of the anterior segment. (c) Full face, showing the dramatic appearance following surgery. The patient is now fully employed. (d) Slit-lamp appearance four years following surgery; the corneal graft remains clear and the AC IOL central. The corneal scar has cleared remarkably.

REFERENCES

1. NHS Executive (2000). *Action on cataracts – Good practice guidance.* HMSO.
2. Desai, P., Minassian, D.C. and Reidy, A. (1999). National Cataract Surgery Survey 1997–8: a report of the results of the clinical outcomes. *Br. J. Ophthalmol.,* **83**, 1336–40.
3. Badoza, D.A., Jure, T., Zunino, L.A. and Argento, C.J. (1999). State-of-the-art phacoemulsification performed by residents in Buenos Aires, Argentina. *J. Cataract Refract. Surg.,* **25**, 1651–5.
4. Cruz, O.A., Wallace, G.W., Gay, C.A., Matoba, A.Y. and Koch, D.D. (1992). Visual results and complications of phacoemulsification with intraocular lens implantation performed by ophthalmology residents. *Ophthalmology,* **99**, 448–52.
5. Desai, P. (1993). National Cataract Surgery Survey II. Clinical outcomes. *Eye,* **7**, 489–94.
6. Prasad, S. (1998). Phacoemulsification learning curve: Experience of two junior trainee ophthalmologists. *J. Cataract Refract.,* **24**, 73–7.
7. Javitt, J.C., Vitale, S., Canner, J.K., Street, D.A., Krakauer, H., McBean, A.M. and Sommer, A. (1991). National outcomes of cataract extraction. Endophthalmitis following inpatient surgery. *Arch. Ophthalmol.,* **109**(8), 1085–9.
8. Schaumberg, D.A., Dana, M.R., Christen, W.G. and Glynn, R.J. (1998). A systematic overview of the incidence of posterior capsule opacification. *Ophthalmology,* **105**, 1213–21.
9. Apple, D.J., Ram, J., Foster, A. and Peng, Q. (2000). Posterior capsule opacification. *Survey of Ophthalmology,* **45**(S1), 100–30.
10. Ram, J., Apple, D.J., Peng, Q., et al. (1999). Update on fixation of rigid and foldable posterior chamber intraocular lenses. Part II. Choosing the correct haptic fixation and intraocular lens design to help eradicate posterior capsule opacification. *Ophthalmology,* **106**, 891–900.
11. Hollick, E.J., Spalton, D.J. and Ursell, P.G. (1999). Surface cytologic features on intraocular lenses; can increased biocompatibility have disadvantages? *Arch. Ophthalmol.,* **117**, 872–8.
12. Ranta, P., Tommila, P., Immonen, I., Summanen, P. and Kivela, T. (2000). Retinal breaks before and after neodymium:YAG posterior capsulotomy. *J. Cataract Refract.,* **26**(8), 1191–7.
13. Olsen, G. and Olson, R.J. (2000). Update on the long term, prospective study of capsulotomy and retinal detachment rates after cataract surgery. *J. Cataract Refract.,* **26**, 1017–21.
14. Nissen, K.R., Fuchs, J., Goldschmidt, E., Andersen, C.U., Bjerum, K., Cory, L., et al. (1998). Retinal detachment after cataract surgery in myopic eyes. *J. Cataract Refract.,* **24**(6), 772–6.
15. Steinert, R.F., Puliafito, C.A., Kumar, S.R., Dudak, S.D. and Patel, S. (1991). Cystoid macula oedema, retinal detachment and glaucoma after Nd:YAG laser posterior capsulotomy. *Am. J. Ophthalmol.,* **112**(4), 373–80.
16. Van Westenbrugge, J.A., Gimbel, H.V., Souchek, J. and Chow, D. (1992). Incidence of retinal detachment following Nd:YAG capsulotomy after cataract surgery. *J. Cataract Refract.,* **18**(4), 352–5.
17. Ficker, L.A., Vickers, S., Capon, M.R., Mellerio, J. and Cooling, R.J. (1987). Retinal detachment following Nd:YAG capsulotomy. *Eye,* **1**(1), 86–9.
18. Albert, D.W., Wade, E.C., Parrish, R.K.II., Flynn, H.W.Jr., Slomovic, A.R., Tanenbaum, M. and Blodi, C. (1990). A prospective study of angiographic cystoid macula oedema one year following Nd:YAG laser posterior capsulotomy. *Ann. Ophthalmol.,* **22**(4), 139–43.
19. Lewis, H., Singer, T.R., Hanscom, T.A. and Straatsma, B.R. (1987). A prospective study of cystoid macula oedema following Nd:YAG laser posterior capsulotomy. *Ophthalmology,* **94**(5), 472–82.
20. Watts, P, Hunter, J and Bunce, C. (2000). Vitrectomy and lensectomy in the management of posterior dislocation of lens fragments. *J. Cataract Refract.,* **26**: 832–7.
21. Borne, M.J., Tasman, W., Rigello, C., et al. (1996). Outcomes of vitrectomy for retained lens fragments. *Ophthalmology,* **103**, 971–6.
22. Bessant, D.A.R., Sullivan, P.M. and Aylward, G.W. (1998). The management of dislocated material after phacoemulsification. *Eye,* **12**, 641–5.
23. Wong, D., Briggs, M.C., Hickey-Dwyer, M.U. and McGalliard, J.N. (1997). Removal of lens fragments from the vitreous cavity. *Eye,* **11**, 37–42.
24. Javitt, J.C., Tielsch, J.M., Canner, J.K., et al. (1992). National outcomes of cataract extraction. Increased risk of retinal complications associated with Nd:YAG laser capsulotomy. *Ophthalmology,* **99**, 1487–97.
25. Norregaard, J.C., Thoning, H., Andersen, T.F., Bernth-Petersen, P. and Javitt, J.C. (1996). Risk of retinal detachment following cataract extraction. Result of the International Cataract Surgery Outcomes Study. *Br. J. Ophthalmol.,* **80**(8), 689–93.
26. Tielsch, J.M., Legro, M.W., Cassard, S.D., et al. (1996). Risk factors for retinal detachment after cataract surgery; a population-based case-control study. *Ophthalmology,* **103**(10), 1537–45.
27. Kanski, J.J. (1994). *Clinical Ophthalmology: A Systemic Approach.* 3rd Edition, Butterworth–Heinemann.
28. Fritch, C.D. (1998). Risk of retinal detachment in myopic eyes after intraocular lens implantation: a 7 year study. *J. Cataract Refract.,* **24**(10), 1357–60.
29. Sasaki, K., Ideta, H., Yonemoto, J., Tanaka, S., Hirose, A. and Oka, C. (1998). Risk of retinal detachment in patients with lattice degeneration. *Jpn. J. Ophthalmol.,* **42**(4), 308–13.
30. Coli, A.F., Price, F.W. and Whitson, W.E. (1993). Intraocular lens exchange for anterior chamber intrao-

cular lens-induced corneal endothelial damage. *Ophthalmology*, **100**: 384–93.

31. Stark, W.J., Gottsch, J.D., Goodman, D.F., Goodman, G.L. and Pratzer, K. (1989). Posterior chamber intraocular lens implantation in the absence of capsular support. *Arch. Ophthalmol.*, **107**, 1078–83.

32. Kraff, M.C., Sanders, D.R., Lieberman H,L., Kraff, J. (1983). Secondary intraocular lens implantation. *Ophthalmology*, **90**, 324–6.

33. Ellerton, C.R., Rattigan, S.M., Chapman, F.M., Chitkara, D.K. and Smerdon, D.L. (1996). Secondary implantation of open-loop, flexible, anterior chamber intraocular lenses. *J Cataract Refract. Surg.*, **22**, 951–4.

34. Navin-Aray, E.A. (1994). Suturing a posterior chamber intraocular lens to the iris through limbal incisions: results in 30 eyes. *J. Cataract Refract. Surg.*, **20**, 565–70.

35. Thompson, C.G., Fawzy, K., Bryce, I.G. and Noble, B.A. Iris sutured intraocular lens implantation in the absence of capsular support. Internal Audit, General Infirmary of Leeds, UK; 1990–1997 (unpublished data).

36. Price, F.W.Jr. and Wellemeyer, M. (1995). Transscleral fixation of posterior chamber intraocular lenses. *J. Cataract Refract. Surg.*, **21**(5), 567–73.

37. McCluskey, P. and Harrisberg, B. (1994). Long-term results using scleral-fixated posterior chamber intraocular lenses. *J. Cataract Refract. Surg.*, **20**(1), 34–9.

38. Lewis, J.S. (1993). Sulcus fixation without flaps. *Ophthalmology*, **100**, 1346–50.

39. Hayward, J.M., Noble, B.A. and George, N. (1990). Secondary lens implantation: eight year experience. *Eye*, **4**, 548–56.

40. Pande, M. and Noble, B.A. (1993). The role of intraocular lens exchange in the management of major implant-related complications. *Eye*, **7**: 34–9.

41. Weene, L.E. (1993). Flexible, open-loop anterior chamber intraocular lens implants. *Ophthalmology*, **100**, 1636–9.

42. Bourke, R.D., Gray, P.J., Rosen, P.H. and Cooling, R.J. (1996). Retinal detachment complicating scleral-sutured posterior chamber intraocular lens surgery. *Eye*, **10**, 501–8.

43. Solomon, K., Gussler, J.R., Gussler, C. and Van Meter, W.S. (1993). Incidence and management of complications of transsclerally sutured posterior chamber lenses. *J. Cataract Refract. Surg,,.* **19**, 488–93.

44. Hennig, A., Evans, J.R., Pradhan, D., et al. (1997). Randomized controlled trial of anterior chamber intraocular lenses. *Lancet,* **349**, 1129–33.

45. Snellingen, T., Shrestha, J.K., Huq, R., et al. (2000). The South Asian cataract study; complication, visual outcomes and corneal endothelial cell loss in a randomized, multi-centre clinical trial comparing intracapsular cataract surgery with and without anterior chamber intraocular lens implantation. *Ophthalmology,* **107**, 231–40.

46. Lim, E.S., Apple, D.J., Tsai, J.C., et al. (1991). An analysis of flexible anterior chamber lenses with special reference to the normalized rate of lens explantation. *Ophthalmology*, **98**, 243–6.

47. Apple, D.J., Ram, J., Foster, A. and Peng, Q. (2000). Anterior chamber intraocular lenses. *Survey of Ophthalmology*, **45**(S1), 131–49.

48. Hu, B.V., Shin, D.H., Gibbs, K.A. and Hong, Y.J. (1988). Implantation of posterior chamber lens in the absence of capsular and zonular support. *Arch. Ophthalmol.*, **106**, 416–20.

49. Schein, O.D., Kenyon, K.R., Steinert, R.F., Verdier, D.D., Waring III, G.O., Stamler, J.F., Seabrook, S.C.O.T. and Vitale, S. (1993). A randomized trial of intraocular lens fixation techniques with penetrating keratoplasty. *Ophthalmology*, **100**, 1437–43.

50. Leon, J.A., Leon, C.S. and Aron-Rosa, D. (2000). Endoscopic technique for suturing posterior chamber intraocular lenses. *J. Cataract Refract. Surg.*, **26**(5), 644–9.

51. The Australian Corneal Graft Registry, 1996 Report. (K.A.Williams, S.M. Muehlberg, R.F. Lewis, L.C. Giles, D.J. Coster, eds). Mercury Press.

52. Burr, J. and Noble, B.A. Internal retrospective audit of 277 PKs perfomed in the General Infirmary of Leeds for the UK corneal graft registry; 1974–1985 (unpublished data).

53. Kirkness, C.M., Ezra, E., Rice, S.C. and McG. Steele, A.D. (1990). The success and survival of repeat corneal grafts. *Eye*, **4**, 58–64.

54. Vail, A., Gore, S.M., Bradley, B.A., Easty, D.L. and Rogers, C.A., on behalf of collaborating surgeons. (1994). Corneal graft survival and visual outcome. *Ophthalmology,* **101**, 120–7.

55. Vail, A., Gore, S.M., Bradley, B.A., Easty, D.L., Rogers, C.A. and Armitage, W.J., on behalf of collaborating surgeons (1997). Conclusions of the corneal transplant follow up study. *Br. J. Ophthalmol.,* **81**, 631–6.

56. Williams, K.A., Roder, D., Esterman, A., Muehlberg, S.M. and Coster, D.J., on behalf of all contributing (1992). Factors predictive of corneal graft survival. Report from the Australian Corneal Graft Registry. *Ophthalmology*, **99**, 403–14.

57. Williams, K.A., Muehlberg, S.M., Lewis, R.F. and Coster, D.J. (1995). How successful is corneal graft transplantation? A report from the Australian Corneal Graft Register. *Eye*, **9**, 219–27.

58. Vail, A., Gore, S.M., Bradley, B.A., Easty, D.L. and Rogers, C.A., on behalf of collaborating surgeons (1993). Corneal transplantation in the United Kingdom and Republic of Ireland. *Br. J. Ophthalmol.,* **77**, 650–6.

59. Volker-Dieben, H.J., Kok-Van Alphen, C.C., Lansbergen, Q. and Persijn, G.G. (1982). Different influences on corneal graft survival in 539 transplants. *Acta Ophthalmol.*, **60**, 190–202.

60. Bishop, V.L.M., Robinson, L.P., Wechsler, A.W. and Billson, F.A. (1986). Corneal graft survival: a retrospective Australian study. *Aust. NZ J. Ophthalmol.*, **14**, 133–8.

61. Sugar, A. (1989). An analysis of corneal endothelial and graft survival in pseudophakic bullous keratopathy. *Trans. Am. Ophthalmol. Soc.,* **87**, 762–801.

62. Olson, R.J., Waltman, S.R., Mattingly, T.P. and Kaufman, H.E. (1979). Visual results after penetrating keratoplasty for aphakic and pseudophakic bullous keratopathy and Fuchs' dystrophy. *Am. J. Ophthalmol.,* **88**, 1000–4.

63. Hassan, T.S., Soong, H.K., Sugar, A. and Meyer, R. (1991). Implantation of Kelman-style open-loop anterior chamber lenses during keratoplasty for aphakic and pseudophakic bullous keratopathy. *Arch. Ophthalmol.,* **98**, 875–80.

64. Koenig, S.B. (1994). Penetrating keratoplasty and intraocular lens exchange: open-loop anterior chamber lenses versus sutured posterior chamber lenses. *Cornea,* **13**(5), 418–21.

65. Soong, H.K., Musch, D.C., Kowal, V., Sugar, A. and Meyer, R.F. (1989). Implantation of posterior chamber intraocular lenses in the absence of lens capsule during penetrating keratoplasty. *Arch. Ophthalmol.,* **107**, 660–5.

66. Desai, P., MacEwen, C.J., Baines, P. and Minassian, C. (1996). Incidence of cases of ocular trauma admitted to hospital and incidence of blinding outcome. *Br. J. Ophthalmol.,* **80**, 592–6.

67. Fong, L.P. (1995). Eye injuries in Victoria, Australia. *Med. J. Aust.,* **162,** 64–8.

68. MacEwen, C.J., Baines, P.S. and Desai, P. (1999). Eye injuries in children: the current picture. *Br. J. Ophthalmol.,* **83**, 933–6.

69. Mulvihill, A. and Eustace, P. (2000). The pattern of perforating eye injuries in Ireland. *Ir. J. Med. Sci.,* **169**(1), 47–9.

70. De Juan Jr., E., Sternberg Jr., P. and Michels, R.G. (1983). Penetrating ocular injuries – types of injuries and visual results. *Ophthalmology,* **90**, 1318–22.

71. Esmaeli, B., Elner, S., Schork, A. and Elner, V. (1995). Predictive factors for the ruptured globe. Visual outcome and ocular survival after penetrating trauma. *Ophthalmology,* **102**, 393–400.

72. Doren, G.S., Cohen, E.J., Brady, S.E., Arentsen, J.J. and Laibson, P.R. (1990). Penetrating keratoplasty after ocular trauma. *Am. J. Ophthalmol.,* **110**, 408–11.

73. Kenyon, K.R., Starck, T. and Hersh, P.S. (1992). Penetrating keratoplasty and anterior segment reconstruction for severe ocular trauma. *Ophthalmology,* **99**, 396–402.

74. Dana, M.R., Schaumberg, D.A., Moyes, A.L., Gomes, J.A,. Laibson, P.R., Holland, E.J., Sugar, A. and Sugar, J. (1995). Outcome of penetrating keratoplasy after ocular trauma in children. *Arch. Ophthalmol.* **113**, 1503–7.

75. Stulting, R.D., Sumers, K.D., Cavanagh, H.D., Waring, G.O. and Gammon, J.A. (1984). Penetrating keratoplasty in children. *Ophthalmology,* **91**, 1222–30.

76. Nobe, J.R., Moura, B.T., Robin, J.B. and Smith, R.E. (1990). Results of penetrating keratoplasty for the treatment of corneal perforations. *Arch. Ophthalmol.,* **108**, 939–41.

77. Groessl, S., Nanda, S.K. and Mieler, W.F. (1993). Assault-related penetrating ocular injury. *Am. J. Ophthalmol.,* **116**, 26–33.

78. Churchill, A.J., Noble, B.A., Etchells, D.E. and George, N.D. (1995). Factors affecting visual outcome following uniocular traumatic cataract. *Eye,* **9**: 285–91.

79. Eckstein, M., Vijayalakshmi, P., Killedar, M., Gilbert, C. and Foster, A. (1998) Use of intraocular lenses in children with traumatic cataract in South India. *Br. J. Ophthalmol.,* **82**, 911–5.

80. Hiles, D.A. (1984). Intraocular lens implantation in children with monocular cataracts. *Ophthalmology,* **91**, 1231–7.

81. Eriksson, A., Koranyi, G., Seregard, S. and Philipson, B. (1998). Risk of acute suprachoroidal haemorrhage with phacoemulsification. *J. Cataract Refract.,* **24**, 793–800.

82. Speaker, M.G., Guerriero, P.N., Met, J.A., et al. (1991). A case-control study of risk factors for intraoperative suprachoroidal expulsive haemorrhage. *Ophthalmology,* **98**, 202–9.

83. Givens, K. and Shields, M.B. (1987). Suprachoroidal haemorrhage after glaucoma filtration surgery. *Am. J. Ophthalmol.,* **103**, 689–94.

84. Price, F.W. Jr., Whitson, M.E., Ahad, K.A. and Tavakkoli, H. (1994). Suprachoroidal haemorrhage in penetrating keratoplasty. *Ophthalmic Surg.,* **25**, 521–5.

Chapter 9

Medical jurisprudence for ophthalmologists

INTRODUCTION

To be able to formulate a strategic approach to reduce the risk of litigation in clinical practice, a surgeon requires a working knowledge of the legal framework that supports his/her profession. Ophthalmology generates only a small percentage of cases that are actually brought to court, hence we must rely on generic legal guidance that has been devised for the medical profession as a whole.

There has been a recent, almost exponential, rise in the risk that a given surgeon will be sued. In 1996, 37 per cent of consultants and senior registrars in the NHS had been sued at least once in their medical careers. The cost to the health service in 1996 to 1997 was around £300 million.

Why is the risk of litigation rising? Probably the most significant reason is that the practice of medicine has become more intrusive. There are more operations available and procedures such as radiological and endoscopic interventions are becoming more frequent. Secondly, the publicity that surrounds miraculous successes and blunders, and the upsurge in medical television dramas, have heightened the public's expectation of cure. Finally, we are living within a 'blame culture'. Accidents no longer happen – an error must have occurred and consequently someone is to blame.

This increasing awareness of the risks of legal challenge affects the doctor, his/her patient and, more importantly, the relationship between the two. Historically, this relationship has been based on morality, which has served to engender trust. The introduction of legal rules has tended to create a more formal and cautious atmosphere as both parties view the other as a potential adversary. As a part of the altruistic NHS, the doctor has been seen in the past as being less financially-driven, hence the popular feeling that he/she has 'done his/her best'. As physicians in general, and surgeons in particular, become increasingly recognized as businessmen, eager to make as much money as possible, the patient population will seek compensation if they feel their investment in health care has been mis-spent.

The legislation on which medical negligence is based is tort law, which is explained in the next section. An understanding of the principles of tort will help you to follow some of the legal arguments and cases that have formed the basis of medico-legal matters in the UK.

WHAT IS TORT LAW?

Tort is part of the law which covers civil wrongs. Where a claimant (C) sues a defendant (D) for a tort, C is complaining that he/she has been a victim of a civil wrong as a consequence of D's actions. A criminal court may 'punish' D for his/her action. A civil court will award monetary 'compensation' to C for any civil wrong done to him/her. The latter is the defining feature of tort law. For example, C is a dental technician working for D. C was sharpening an instrument on a grinder when a piece flew into his eye. D was found liable for the injury as she did not issue safety goggles and did not enforce their use.

Tort law covers the wrong-doings of defamation, trespass and nuisance. D can also be held responsible for his/her animals and his/her employees. An array of careless behaviour, which might threaten C's person or property, may constitute the tort of negligence.

Negligence broadly means that D's actions have been sufficiently careless to lead to a compromise in C's interests. It needs to be shown, however, if D needs to be concerned with C's interests at all and if so, 'how concerned' he/she should be. In legal terms, the former equates to a duty of care and the latter to a standard of care. In general, if C wishes to prove negligence against D, he/she must show that D owed him/her a duty of care, that the duty of care was breached 'and that loss resulted'.

The origins of the 'duty of care' in medicine dates back to religious leaders and philosophers. In the Western world, Christianity and Judaism dictated the moral basis on which the majority of medical ethics is founded. In ancient Greece, the philosopher Hippocrates set out a code of conduct that superseded that previously suggested by the religious fraternity. The resulting Hippocratic Oath was recently updated and provides the basis for an International Code of Medical Ethics. Interestingly, the concept of a 'duty of care' has no legal consequences until it is broken.

Why does tort law exist? Tort should deter and thus prevent D damaging C in the first place. It should also provide a remedy to the wrong-doing in terms of monetary compensation. The trouble is that in a significant number of medical cases, money does not appear to be the answer. Many claimants are often after an explanation or an apology. When these are not forthcoming, we should not be surprised by their pursuance of financial recompense as that is all that is on offer. Defendants, often health authorities responsible for their employees, complain that the money for negligence cases comes out of the same pot as that used to treat other patients. The higher the damages, the less provision afforded to the remaining health community.

MEDICAL JURISPRUDENCE IN THE UK

In the eighteenth century, the practice of medicine in Britain would have seemed very corrupt by today's standards. Medical ethics was overshadowed by the drive for fame, fortune and academic recognition. In an attempt to restore a code of practice to the profession, the British Medical Association (BMA) was founded in 1832. This was, and always has been, a self-governing body, which today is a non-affiliated registered trade union for doctors. There needed to be an independent body capable of objective scrutiny that would have the respect of the lay population. The General Medical Council (GMC) was established by the Medical Act 1858. Its basic functions are to maintain an official register of medical practitioners, to oversee medical education and to dictate the standards of fitness to practice. The Professional Conduct Committee (PCC) is the ultimate tribunal for doctors accused of misconduct. Appeal against rulings from this body are heard by the Privy Council.

Historically, there has been criticism of the GMC in that 'peer control' provides an inadequate protection for the public. The Medical (Professional Performance) Act of 1995 has forced the GMC to become responsible for the technical ability of the practitioners it has registered.

WHO IS TO BLAME – WHOM DO I SUE?

Medical negligence

Much as all drivers are legally obliged to take out insurance, before 1990 all doctors were contractually bound to subscribe to a defence organization (e.g. the Medical Defence Union or Medical Protection Society). As subscription rates increased dramatically, it was decided that it was financially more viable for NHS indemnity to be extended to doctors, dentists and community physicians. From 1990, therefore, the entire costs of negligence litigation has been borne by the NHS. As a result of this, health authorities may now feel that it makes better economical sense to admit liability, to settle rather than contest a claim, which may not be the fairest option for the physician concerned. NHS indemnity will not cover work outside of the NHS, which will include private practice, 'good Samaritan' work and medico-legal reports.

NEGLIGENCE

The claimant in any action must prove, on the balance of probabilities, that the standard of medical care given fell below that expected by the law, i.e. there was 'fault', in the legal sense of the word. How this should be achieved is covered below but the current system is loaded towards the defendant. Only a small proportion of victims of medical negligence will sue and of those cases over 80 per cent will fail. However, with increasing public awareness, the number of claims is rising. Even if successful, the plaintiff may have to wait three or more years before receiving their compensation. This has sparked an argument for the UK to introduce the New Zealand system of 'no-fault' compensation.

Dissatisfaction with the medico-legal system is almost universal. New protocols introduced as a part of the recent Woolf reforms were intended to and may increase the efficiency and appropriateness of medical litigation. Time will tell. In practice, proof of causation is much more difficult, costly and time-consuming than proof of fault.

How does the law set the standard of medical care that should be offered? The answer to this question forms the basis of the 'Bolam test' of medical competence. It is derived from a ruling in a sentinel case: *Bolam vs Friern Hospital Management Committee* (1957) as slightly modified by the case of *Sidaway vs Board of Governors of the Bethlehem Royal and Maudsley Hospital* (1985).

The test is the standard of the ordinary skilled physician exercising and professing to have that special skill. A physician need not possess the highest expert skill at the risk of being found negligent. It is a well-established law that 'it is sufficient if he/she exercises the ordinary skill of an ordinary [physician] exercising that particular art'. A doctor is not guilty of negligence if he/she has acted in accordance with a practice rightly accepted as proper by a responsible body of medical men skilled in that particular art. Putting it another way, a physician is not negligent if he/she is acting in accordance with such a practice, merely because there is a body of opinion which would take a contrary view.

Subsequent cases have actually taken things further by decreeing that a 'mere error of judgement' is not necessarily negligence, even if its results are catastrophic.

Although the 'Bolam test' survives, it has its critics. The standard of care expected is that of a doctor practising with the degree of competence of the ordinary skilful physician. The more skills a specialist possesses, the higher the standard of care expected. How does the law dictate where the dividing line sits between ordinary and above/below this mark? The law is directed by representation from the medical profession. To the public, this must seem like the epitome of rank-closing.

Accidental trauma

Injuries occurring in the home, at the workplace and on public property are becoming less 'accidental'. Even if the victim was solely responsible, blame is often sought elsewhere. Television and newspaper advertisements advise all victims to contact legal firms to identify whom should be sued. Not only the manufacturer, but also those who assemble and repair the tools and objects concerned, may be liable for injury caused by a particular product. In general, cases where legal action will be successful are where the consumer has been injured despite using the product in a responsible way.

The standard of care is different if at home or at work. A grinder may come with a written warning for use at home; goggles may be advised for use. If the victim ignores the warning and suffers an eye injury by not wearing protective glasses, the victim has no one to blame but him/herself. If, however, he/she is at work using the same machine, his/her employers might have a legal duty of care to supply safety goggles and ensure their use. The fact that the machine came with a written warning is no defence, as the victim may not have read it.

The Employers' Liability (Defective Equipment) Act 1969 provides that the employer is liable for equipment which is defective through the negligence of third parties. If the goggles, provided by the employer and worn by the employee, shatter whilst in use because of a faulty protective coating, the employer, not the goggles manufacturer, is liable for the resulting injury. The employer might then sue the goggles manufacturer but this would be a separate legal suit.

The rest of this chapter will be primarily devoted to the discussion of negligence issues within medical care.

WHAT CONSTITUTES ACCEPTABLE PRACTICE?

To be able to show that a physician has departed from 'usual and normal practice', the claimant must show that there is a rightly accepted 'usual and normal practice' (dictated by guidelines that are drawn up by the Royal College of Ophthalmologists for eye surgeons in the UK), that the physician has not adopted it and that the course that was chosen would not have been taken by the ordinary ophthalmologist acting with ordinary care.

Such usual and normal practice will be pursued by a significant body of the profession. Research in ophthalmology is moving forwards at a considerable pace. Should we be aware of all the current theories as to the ways we should treat our patients? The legal position is that a physician should not be held as negligent if he/she has not read a particular article or has not put the knowledge from that article into practice. He/she is negligent if a series of warnings in the medical press have all been ignored or if he/she has failed to advance his/her practice in line with the majority of his/her colleagues.

'Usual and normal practice' can be applied to diagnoses. A mistake in diagnosis will not be deemed negligent if the other aspects of care fall within the standard expected. If, however, the reason for the misdiagnosis was that the doctor failed to take a proper history, failed to perform a thorough examination or failed to order the appropriate investigations, then the doctor could be considered culpable.

The most important distinction in determining whether treatment has been negligent is between a medical mistake, which the law can excuse, and a mistake which would amount to negligence. An example of the former might be rupturing the posterior capsule during phaco surgery. An example of the latter might be operating on the wrong eye. In any operation, it is the surgeon's responsibility to use an instrument in or around the eye and it is his/her responsibility to subsequently remove it, if appropriate. To say 'I relied on the nurse to tell me how many needles I had used' cannot be used in absolution of mistakenly leaving one in the eye.

HOW DOES THE LAW TREAT TRAINEES?

A newly appointed trainee will not have the surgical experience of a senior consultant, so reason would have it that less should be expected of the former – he/she should be given leeway. That is not the way the law sees things. The strict application of Bolam demands that the treatment of any physician should be compared, in an objective way, to the legal standard of care expected, no matter what his/her experience. Having said that, the required standard of care is very likely to be met if the junior member of staff seeks senior advice at an appropriate time. Delegation of responsibility to a junior may, in itself, constitute negligence. A consultant would be liable if he/she delegated a duty that he/she knew the junior was unable to perform.

As a trainer you will appreciate the junior member of staff who knows his/her own abilities and limitations – a trainee with insight. It is your responsibility, however, to know these abilities and limitations yourself so that only appropriate work is delegated downwards.

RES IPSA LOQUITUR

It can sometimes be very difficult for the victim of negligent medical care to identify who or what is to blame. Whereas it is usually up to C to prove that D has broken the duty of care, C can invoke the doctrine of 'Res ipsa loquitur' which means literally 'the matter speaks for itself'. The implication is that the facts point towards D's culpability so much that it is D's onus to offer an alternative explanation. For example, if C ends up after anterior segment surgery with a needle in his/her eye, he/she may be sufficiently unaware of the surgical procedure to know who to blame. The surgeon would therefore have to show that he/she exercised care to ensure that a needle was not left in the eye.

CAUSATION

As we have shown, the problems of proving fault in cases of medical negligence are significant. On top of these, however, it is pointless proving negligence if the claimant cannot show that the damage he/she has suffered was caused by that negligence.

The starting point in causation is the assumption that C would not have suffered the injury 'but for' D's tort. (This is sometimes called the 'but for test'.) It has been held that where there is a precaution that could have been taken to prevent the very injury suffered, the onus will revert to D to establish that his/her failure to take this precaution did not lead to C's injury (a type of res ipsa loquitur). The problem comes where there are a number of possibilities for a cause of the injury. For example, C may claim that by not cleaning the eye with povidone–iodine, D had caused postoperative endophthalmitis. D may contend that the instruments may have been contaminated or that the theatre air was unclean. The onus of proof lies with the claimant.

The 'but for test' runs into problems where it is unclear what would have happened if D had not committed the tort. For example, if a surgeon implants the wrong IOL but that patient has also got diabetic maculopathy, the claim for damage to sight may be tempered by the long-term prognosis of patients with diabetic eye disease. To a victim of medical negligence, this approach will seem grossly biased towards the defendant surgeon who is often given the benefit of the doubt.

Factual uncertainty

An 80-year-old lady presented to the accident and emergency department having fallen in the street. She had a progressively worsening proptosis and bruising around her eye. The ophthalmic registrar was called but he did not attend. The retro-bulbar haemorrhage led to permanent optic neuropathy and a vision of counting fingers in a previously healthy eye. The registrar's defence was that, tak-

ing into account his travelling time, he would have been at the patient's bedside three hours after the initial fall and thus his presence, or his intervention, would have had no effect on the final visual acuity. The resulting compressive optic neuropathy would have caused irreversible damage. The court held that there was no liability because any negligence was not causative of her injury: if the registrar had complied with his duty of care (attending the patient) the lady would still have gone blind. Here there was factual uncertainty about the end result, either with or without the undelivered care.

Factual uncertainty has been used in defence of D in cases of accidental trauma. It may be possible to show that wearing protective goggles would have prevented C's eye injury. D might be able to show, however, that from previous experience, C would have been unlikely to wear the goggles even if they were provided. C may have turned down the opportunity to use protective equipment in the past. If this was held, there would be no causal connection between his/her employer's breach of duty and C's ocular injury.

The 'thin-skull' rule

Where D is held to be negligent in inflicting damage on C and then, because of some pre-existing condition, the damage becomes more extensive than first imagined, D is liable for it all. This is the 'thin skull' rule. An example in ophthalmology might be the surgeon who decided to implant too small an anterior chamber lens in an eye with Fuchs' endothelial dystrophy. Whereas the tort may not have led to pseudophakic bullous keratopathy, needing a corneal graft, in a normal eye, it did in the eye that had a predisposition to this problem. D, if found liable, would be responsible for the further corneal surgery that might be required.

CONSENT

Any surgery we perform on our patients is a form of legalized assault. This assault is only deemed legal if the patient has consented to the operation.

C can bring an action for battery if he/she has been touched by D in the absence of express or implied consent. All that needs to be established is that D touched C whether or not damage or loss has ensued. It is an appropriate course of action if the surgery performed was completely unconnected with the procedure that C consented to or where there was no consent at all. An example of the former would be a patient who had undergone a dacryocystorhinostomy where he/she had, in fact, consented to cataract surgery.

If a patient undergoes an operation but the consent is flawed, then the appropriate course of action will be that based on the tort of negligence. Consent can be deemed to be flawed if there is a failure to disclose risk. For an action based on negligence to succeed, C must show that D wrongfully touched him/her and that by doing so, an injury resulted. In this scenario, there is a problem of factual causation to be addressed. It will be apparent that an action for battery is an easier option for C, if the circumstances allow for it.

By claiming the surgeon was negligent in obtaining consent, C is saying, 'You did not inform me of the risks of the procedure. If I had known about these I would not have consented to the operation. You have failed in your duty of care and I have sustained damage because of your failings'. A patient suffering an expulsive haemorrhage during cataract surgery will undoubtedly wish they had never consented for the operation in the first place. He/she may thus claim that he/she was insufficiently informed about the potential risks. The question remains, however, would that patient have still consented to the procedure even if the risks had been thoroughly explained? How does the law decide whether consent has been sufficient?

The courts can postulate what a hypothetical reasonable patient, invested with the pertinent clinical and social situation, would do if faced with the risks of surgery. Would that patient have consented to the proposed operation? If the patient with the expulsive haemorrhage saw only 6/60 in both eyes and had a disabled wife/husband, the court might argue that a reasonable patient would consent for surgery 'despite' all the risks.

Of note, whilst there is a proven need for a patient to have given his/her consent, there is no legal basis for a patient to 'demand' treatment. This 'gift' lies entirely with the doctor.

Informed consent

The term 'informed consent' was first used in English law in the early 1980s, whereas it was initially coined in America in the late 1950s. The inferred definition is that a patient should only be operated upon if he/she knows the risks of that surgery and consents to the procedure in this knowledge. It follows that he/she cannot be expected to make a decision, which is based on risk, without the relevant factual information. This begs the following question: 'What constitutes an acceptable standard of information, both in terms of breadth and depth?'

There are two standards of information disclosure: patient and professional. For the former, the doctor must disclose all the relevant facts. It is not for the doctor to decide what the patient should and should not hear. There is obviously a risk that excessive information might confuse or distress the patient, hence the courts will usually accept a degree of therapeutic privilege where the information might be reduced. In determining whether consent has been adequate, the courts will consider if the information disclosed was sufficient for a 'reasonable patient' to make a decision.

A 'professional standard' for information disclosure considers counselling within clinical management and is thus a matter for the attending physician. The information offered by the physician will be compared to that offered by a 'reasonable doctor' when the court decides if there has been a breach of the duty of care in obtaining consent.

With the constraints of time in the NHS, and possibility of unnecessarily disturbing the patient, the courts will tend to follow the professional standard. The added advantage of this approach is that clearer guidelines can be laid down allowing for objective judicial consistency.

Although there is no clear basis in law, reason would have it that we owe a duty to our patients to ensure they 'understand' the risks of surgery, rather than simply disclosing information. As we mentioned in Chapter 1, a patient is more likely to accept a poor outcome if they understood the risks of surgery pre-operatively. The doctor–patient relationship will be harder to maintain if, despite pages of A4 literature, the patient still claims he/she did not fully comprehend the risks.

What constitutes a negligible risk?

Various percentage risks are bandied around concerning informed consent. Some surgeons maintain they only have to warn a patient if the risk of a potential complication is above 5 per cent. Some say this figure should be 2 per cent. UK law refers back to Bolam, in this instance, where a particular doctor will 'not be considered negligent if he/she acts in accordance with a practice accepted at the time as proper by a responsible body of medical opinion'. In other words a reasonably prudent doctor would inform a patient of a risk if it was so obviously necessary to make an informed decision.

A risk should be considered significant or material if a reasonable person, in the patient's position, if warned of that risk, would attach significance to it. If a patient asks questions specifically about that risk, it is logical to assume that he/she attaches significance to it. If a patient asks about the risks of losing sight altogether following cataract surgery, it would therefore be negligent not to inform him/her of the possibility of endophthalmitis and suprachoroidal haemorrhage even though the risks are below 1 in 1000.

Efficient information disclosure

The path to a patient's understanding of the risks of surgery, which will form the basis of informed consent, can be circuitous and drawn-out. Below is a suggested approach to informing a patient of the risks of cataract surgery (you will need to substitute your own audit figures for the ones marked with an asterisk):

'In about 95 per cent* of cases, patients will notice a visual improvement, provided the rest of the eye is healthy. The most common major complication is rupture of the posterior capsule, the bag in which your cataract lies and the new implant will sit. In my hands this occurs in 2 per cent* of cases. Vision may well be better despite this complication. Less common, but more serious, complications include infection and haemorrhage. In these cases vision can be worse than before surgery and may be lost altogether.'

If a patient wants to know more details he/she will ask you and you then have a duty to inform, even if the risks he/she is asking about are very uncommon. By grouping the potential risks in headings you will have complied with your duty of care and have given the patient an opportunity to ask questions if more information is required.

PERSONAL INJURY DAMAGES

How is compensation paid?

Negligence has been proved. In tort law, C is now entitled to compensation. How is this calculated? The inherent problem with a monetary remedy is that it will never accurately compensate for non-pecuniary loss, for example, loss of vision, chronic ocular pain, enjoyment of life, etc. Even where it should be easier, e.g. calculating loss of income, it is ultimately impossible to have predicted what would have happened if the tort had not occurred.

Very few cases actually come to court. Most settlements are reached between the lawyers acting for C and D. The process is not a quick one – the average delay being upwards of 20 months. This seems to unfairly penalize C who may have to rely on sickness benefit and the social security system. Where liability is not an issue, claimants can apply for interim payment of damages prior to the conclusion of the case. In general, the defendants are large corporate bodies, hospitals or health authorities with respect to medical negligence, and employers or manufacturers in the field of ocular trauma. This is a double-edged sword for C. D's legal team will be able to drive damage settlements down but ultimately D will be able to afford to pay.

Damages are usually awarded in a lump sum. There are two main components: a sum to compensate for the injury and its non-pecuniary consequences and a sum to compensate for direct financial losses which will include future expenses such as loss of earnings. Where there will be recurrent loss, e.g. salary, the court will calculate the estimated net loss for a typical year (the 'multiplicand'). This amount will then be adjusted for the number of years that will be affected (by using a 'multiplier'). The multiplier will usually appear very low at first glance but takes account of the acceleration of payment, so C is expected to invest the lump sum which will then appreciate with interest, and the 'exigencies of life'. At present the courts assume that interest will be accrued at a rate of 3 per cent per annum and will adjust the lump sum accordingly.

How is the victim of the tort assessed?

Personal injury damages are calculated under the following headings:

(1) Pain, suffering and loss of amenity, i.e. compensation for the injury and its non-financial consequences.

(2) Loss of earnings.

(3) Past and future expenses.

PAIN, SUFFERING AND LOSS OF AMENITY

'Pain and suffering' damages compensate for the nature of the injury and the suffering caused by it. 'Loss of the amenities of life' damages compensate for its non-financial affects (e.g. being unable to continue a hobby, pastime or a particularly satisfying job). A single sum is usually awarded for both of these losses without subdividing the remedy under the two subheadings. Clear guidelines are provided for judges by the Guidelines for the Assessment of General Damages in Personal Injury Cases published (and regularly updated) by the Judicial Studies Board, summarized in Table 9.1.

LOSS OF EARNINGS

Net earnings lost before settlement have to be estimated on the basis of expected income and require documentary proof. They can then be dealt with as 'special damages'. Future loss of earnings are then calculated on the above multiplicand–multiplier basis. C may claim the multiplicand should be increased to account for the prospects of promotion: D may contend the multiplier should be reduced to reflect the possibility of redundancy.

Sometimes the courts have to award damages for 'loss of earning capacity', to reflect the loss of a possibility to enter more remunerative employment as a result of the injury. A typical case would be a young boy who lost his sight in both eyes. Provision needs to be made for recognition of the fact that the types of work available to him/her in adulthood will be severely restricted by his disability, so he/she will be more vulnerable on the open labour market than most others.

PAST AND FUTURE EXPENSES

Past expenses are those incurred between the injury and the date of the settlement/trial and are easily assessed. Future recurring expenses are usually also calculated on a multiplicand–multiplier basis. C can only recover costs of 'reasonable' expenses but these can be extensive. For instance a patient can decide to be treated privately. This is not deemed 'unreasonable' just because a similar service

Table 9.1. Guidelines for the assessment of ocular damage in personal injury cases.

(a) Total blindness and deafness	£200 000
(b) Total blindness	£135 000
(c) Loss of sight in one eye with reduced vision in the remaining eye	
Where there is a serious risk of further deterioration in the remaining eye, going beyond some risk of sympathetic ophthalmia	£48 000–£90 000
Where there is reduced vision in the remaining eye and/or additional problems such as double vision	£32000–£53 000
(d) Total loss of one eye	£28 000–£33 000
The level of the award within the bracket will depend on age and cosmetic effect	
(e) Complete loss of sight in one eye	£25 000–£28 000
This award takes account of some risk of sympathetic ophthalmia. The upper end of the bracket is appropriate where there is scarring in the region of the eye which is not sufficiently serious to merit a separate award.	
(f) Cases of serious but incomplete loss of vision in one eye without significant risk of loss or reduction of vision in the remaining eye, or where there is constant double vision.	£12 000–£20 000
(g) Minor but permanent impairment of vision in one eye, including cases where there is some double vision, which may not be constant	£6 250–£10 500
(h) Minor eye injuries	£2 000–£4 250
In this bracket fall cases of minor injuries, such as being struck in the eye, exposure to fumes including smoke, or being splashed by liquids, causing initial pain and some interference with vision, but no lasting effects.	
(i) Transient eye injuries	£1 000–£2 000
In these cases the injured person will have recovered completely within a few weeks.	

is available on the NHS. Similarly, claims may be made for the cost of employing contractors to perform domestic tasks previously undertaken by C, e.g. gardening, decorating, etc.

THE LITIGIOUS PATIENT

There is no defining characteristic that identifies the patient who will sue, but there is one emotion that links all litigious patients and that is anger. Most patients seek medical care because they want to be cured not because they are thinking of suing. With the recent advances in medical care, patients not only want to be cured, they 'expect' to be cured. When these expectations are not realized some will seek litigation as redress. Surprise at a poorer than expected outcome may turn to anger if communication between the surgeon and patient is poor or avoided.

Good patient education in the pre-operative work-up is the physician's chance to ground expectation in realism. If a complication occurs, the doctor–patient relationship will be tested. The stronger it is, the better the chance of helping the patient over a difficult period. If there are problems and issues that cannot be rapidly resolved, it is often best to pre-empt matters and offer the patient a second opinion with another expert. Time should be set aside which can be devoted to post-operative counselling. The patient should be seen regularly by the most senior member of the team in clinic. Openness and honesty will foster trust.

WHICH CASES END UP IN COURT?

Any problem that results in a less than perfect functional and cosmetic result can generate a medico-legal claim. Most litigation following cataract surgery is due to mistakes with the IOL. Inaccurate biometry, failing to take into account the refractive state of the fellow eye and problems reading a written note can all lead to the wrong power being used. This may require a contact lens, refractive surgery, 'piggybacking' or IOL exchange to correct. Decentration or malposition of an IOL can cause just as many subjective problems.

Any surgical complication can result in legal proceedings but the most common are those which lead to a poorer visual outcome. These will include a ruptured posterior capsule, vitreous loss and retained lens material. Expulsive haemorrhage and endophthalmitis are the complications we most fear, as they result in the worst visual outcome or even loss of an eye.

Provided the patient did not have uncontrolled hypertension or poor blood clotting secondary to warfarin, suprachoroidal haemorrhage is easy to defend. Fewer of the ensuing problems can be attributed to the surgeon.

Conversely, endophthalmitis cases are usually the most expensive as it is easier to blame the surgeon for lack of vigilance or incomplete pre- and post-operative management. The usual complaint in these cases is that while post-operative inflammation was noted, it was not aggressively investigated or treated. Factual uncertainty may be contested by D as the exact cause for the infection may be difficult to establish (see above).

A well-managed complication may result in a good visual outcome, which makes litigation less likely. The main reason any case, whether surgical or medical, ends up in court is a breakdown of the doctor–patient relationship which usually stems from a lack of honesty and openness by the clinician.

RISK-REDUCTION STRATEGIES

There are some management strategies and protocols that can be followed which reduce the risk of an adverse event and subsequent litigation. Some of these strategies can be applied to all ophthalmic procedures and some are specifically for cataract surgery. These are set out in Tables 9.2 and 9.3, respectively.

The singular most important device to prevent litigation is communication. This needs to be comprehensive and must be seen/documented to be so. Medical records should

Table 9.2. General ophthalmic risk reduction.

- Fully document the pre-operative examination, especially noting positive and negative findings which may affect outcome, and the indications for surgery.
- Document the discussion concerning risks of surgery and prognosis.
- Indicate if an education sheet/booklet has been given to the patient.
- Obtain informed consent – the use of an operation-specific consent form will help.
- Write or dictate a complete operative report. This should include any steps to prevent infection (povidone-iodine wash, intracameral or post-operative antibiotics), the description of any complication and the steps taken to manage it and the reasons for choosing a particular IOL power and style. Document the absence of complications and the use of various preparations, no matter how routine.
- Take all patients' concerns seriously after the operation.
- Manage all flashes, floaters, pain and visual deterioration aggressively.
- Afford more time to follow up patients who are angry or aggrieved. Discussions should be thoroughly documented and, preferably, witnessed.
- Never make any changes to a previous record on the basis of belatedly observed findings.
- Ask for senior advice or a second opinion early.

Table 9.3. Risk reduction in cataract surgery.

- Ensure technicians or nurses who perform biometry are well-trained.
- Review the A-scans and other data yourself.
- Use a third-generation formula for IOL power calculation.
- Use a limited number of IOL styles to prevent confusion and have their A-constants pinned to the side of their cabinet.
- Clearly mark the IOL power and style on an operating list in the theatre either on a white board or on paper.
- Do not operate beyond your experience, e.g. don't try to remove a dropped nuclear fragment or attempt a complicated lens implant unless you have been shown how.

be seen as the physician's best ally, although they may often be our worst enemy.

SCALES OF COMPENSATION IN OPHTHALMOLOGY

In assessing the impact of ocular damage, the courts have relied on a report produced in 1958 under the chairmanship of Dr Leon Hambresin, entitled 'An Attempt to Standardize the Scales of Compensation in Ophthalmology'. This report attempted to obtain uniformity with regards to compensation rates awarded when an eye is damaged or becomes impaired functionally. It takes into account the scales granted in different countries in North America, Europe and Australasia. Before this report was presented, guidelines were scarce for the ophthalmologist in the field of compensation. An overview of this report, with information relevant to this book, is now presented.

In terms of visual loss, the eye is considered blind if Snellen acuity is less than 3/60, as at this level there is insufficient vision in that eye for working purposes. This reflects the level of vision set by the National Assistance Act of 1948 in the UK for eligibility to be registered blind. It was suggested that this be the lower limit of working vision and that the upper limit, i.e. the level of vision below which compensation should be awarded, be set at 6/12. In doing this, however, one needed to consider the ability of that person to earn a salary in pursuing not only his/her own occupation but any occupation.

In suggesting the scales of compensation, the general principles agreed on were that loss of vision from both eyes represented a more significant defect as not only can the person not work, but immediately loses his/her ability to be independent. In addition, any injury that results in (cosmetic) disfigurement should be compensated, as it would undoubtedly affect his/her capacity to compete in a job. Percentage losses are presented below and are summarized in Table 9.4.

Compensation rates

BLINDNESS

Where vision is completely (both eyes) lost, 100 per cent compensation should be awarded.

LOSS OF VISION IN ONE EYE WITH THE OTHER BEING NORMAL

Twenty-seven per cent if there is no disfigurement, 30 per cent with disfigurement.

LOSS OF EYEBALL

Thirty per cent if permitting prosthesis, 35 per cent if a prosthesis is not possible and 40 per cent if a prosthesis is not possible with serious disfigurement.

REDUCTION OF VISION OF ONE OR BOTH EYES
(see Table 9.4)

The vision should be that with correction and if there is intolerance to the refractive device, the compensation should be increased by 3 per cent.

CONCENTRIC LOSS OF VISUAL FIELD

Unilateral down to 20 degrees:	5%
Unilateral to less than 10 degrees:	12%
Bilateral down to 20 degrees:	20%
Bilateral to less than 10 degrees:	80%

CENTRAL SCOTOMA

Unilateral:	25% maximum
Bilateral:	100% maximum

HEMIANOPIA

Homonymous:	35%	
Heteronymous:	Bitemporal:	20%
	Binasal:	10%
Altitudinal defects:	Upper:	20%
	Lower:	60%
Quadrantic defects:	Homonymous upper:	10%
	Homonymous lower:	25%
	Heteronymous upper temporal:	6%
	Heteronymous lower temporal:	14%
	Heteronymous upper nasal:	3%
	Heteronymous lower nasal:	7%

HEMIANOPIA IN A ONE-EYED PERSON

Defect in nasal field:	40%
Defect in temporal field:	50%
Defect in upper visual field:	25%
Defect in lower visual field:	65%

DIPLOPIA

If requiring occlusion of an eye   22%
If occlusion not required, depending on the degree of deficiency and whether double vision is in the upper or lower visual field: 5–17%

APHAKIA

Unilateral

(1) If the phakic eye has working vision with or without correction: 18 per cent, plus one-third of the rate given in the valuation table.
(2) If the phakic eye does not have working vision with or without correction, but has an acuity equal or better than that of the aphakic eye: 18 per cent, plus the rate given in the valuation table, not exceeding 100 per cent.
(3) If the aphakic eye has better vision than the phakic eye with or without correction and the aphakic eye is used to see: 21 per cent, plus the rate given in the valuation table, not exceeding 100 per cent.

Bilateral

Thirty per cent, plus the rate given in the valuation table, not exceeding 100 per cent.

Table 9.4. Valuation table of scales of compensation (as adapted from Hambresin).

	6/6–6/9	6/12	6/18	6/24	6/36	6/60	4/60	3/60	0 (NPL)
% compensation									
6/6–6/9	0	0	5	10	10	15	20	20	25
6/12	0	5	10	10	15	25	25	30	35
6/18	5	10	25	25	30	35	40	45	55
6/24	10	10	25	40	40	50	55	60	65
6/36	10	15	30	40	55	65	70	75	80
6/60	15	25	35	50	65	85	90	95	105
4/60	20	25	40	55	70	90	95	100	115
3/60	20	30	45	60	75	95	100	110	125
0 (NPL)	25	35	55	65	80	105	115	125	125

COLOBOMA OF THE IRIS/IRIDODIALYSIS

Compensation if breach lies in the lower half of the iris: 2%
If there is monocular diplopia: 3–5%.

MYDRIASIS, ALONE AND CAUSING FUNCTIONAL DISTURBANCE

Unilateral: 5%
Bilateral: 10%

Index